I Left My Heart
At Stanford . . .

But They Gave Me
A New One

by

Don & Mary Coover

Published by Arrowhead Classics Publishing
P O Box 1247
Newcastle, California
http://www.arrowhead-classics.com

First Edition: January, 2013

For more about the authors see the last page of this book.

ISBN:1481045679
Cataloging in Publications Data
Coover, Don
1. Heart Transplant - Health.

10 9 8 7 6 5 4 3 2 1

Index

Preface

After Don Coover successfully survived two heart transplants and one kidney transplant, he and his wife sat down and wrote about their experience of living through a frightening period together.

Each chapter in this book offers a perspective from Don or Mary of the progression of Don's life-saving transplants.

It is a story for others who might be entering the same long tunnel, especially since there is a light at the other end and it reflects a happy ending.

— Donald Gazzaniga
Megaheart.com

1
Beginning Years

Don

The last thing I remembered while being wheeled into surgery at Stanford University Hospital in Palo Alto, California was my wife Mary saying, "Think sex." These were her parting words before my many surgeries that I was to experience in my adult life. These surgeries would be the result of health issues from birth.

On October 31, 1944, I was born six weeks prematurely at Santa Rosa's Tanner Hospital and weighed only three pounds. The hospital was housed in what was once an old Victorian home. I was delivered by Dr. Alexis Maximov, who was one of the first OB/GYN specialists in the area. He asked one of the attending nurses if he could borrow her hot water bottle which she had brought to work for her stomach cramps. Dr. Maximov placed me in a shoe box with the hot water bottle under my tiny and wrinkled body for transportation in his car to County Hospital, which was north of town and where they had incubators. Hospitals in those days were far from what we have today, especially in a small town, which Santa Rosa, California was then. I remained at County Hospital for approximately six weeks until I was strong enough for going home. With being premature, my lungs and digestive system were not fully developed. So having that six week stay was very important for helping my little body get a decent start in life. Having a Halloween birthday and with being born surprisingly prematurely, I don't know, even to this day, whether I was a trick or a treat. Maybe neither or maybe both.

I learned that being born prematurely was just the beginning of a very interesting and challenging childhood and an adult life full of surprises. I had tender skin which would cut, tear, and traumatize easily. As a child, I knew early on that I was different from the other children. I would fall as most kids do, however a cut or a scrape on most children would end up being a gash on me, whether it be on an arm or leg or even torso. The injury would be a gaping wound requiring hours of stitching and butterfly closures. Ending up in the emergency room or the doctor's office was a rather common occurrence, with follow-up visits, possibly for weeks during the healing process. The wound would not bleed much, however the skin would tear and separate as though there was no skin there to begin with. Through my younger years, I had to be very careful, trying to avoid rough physical contact while playing with friends and participating in sporting activities. However, that did not always work out as planned, and I have the battle scars to this day as evidence. Some examples through childhood and into my adult years were; falling off monkey bars and splitting open my chin, falling off the bicycle and ripping open my side on the bike chain, slipping off the bike pedals and tearing open the back of my calf above the ankle, and splitting open the inside of my calf while falling through the steps of bleachers at a football game. I also split open the inside of my left calf in the process of falling off the roof of my parent's house and into the bushes below while helping with a re-roofing job. Another time involved ripping open the back of my calf as I slipped on a wet step of the front porch. You might think I was a klutz and should have lived in a plastic bubble, but as I mentioned before, my hyper-elastic skin was the culprit.

My father was a big man with skin like cow hide and he played all sports well, through high school and college, earning a football scholarship. Athletics were an important part of his formative years, so I felt I had a need for trying to follow in his footsteps. I played Little League Baseball and tried basketball and track. Although, it didn't take long to realize I was not able to be as aggressive as was needed for excelling in those activities. I always had a fear of injuring myself when it came to contact sports, so I settled on swimming which gave me a better chance of avoiding bruising and tearing open my skin. I felt safe in the swimming pool, spending summers on a community pool team and three years competing on my high school team. While the other spring sport athletes were sweating on the track or the baseball diamond, all of us swimmers were nice and cool in the pool.

While growing up I never knew of any other children that had my skin condition. Believing at the time, it was only a skin problem and with proper precautions, I thought I was able to live a good quality of life. I was somewhat of a side show growing up. I could pull my skin several inches away from my body, especially at the joints, knees, elbows, neck, and underside of the arms. The term, "chicken skin" could have been a good comparison. Kids would call me Stretch. I guess I thought it was kind of fun. I could also flip my upper eyelids up and make my fingers and thumbs bend into right angles.

I lived into my 40s thinking my situation was just a hyper-elastic skin condition. However, by my mid-40s, I started to develop heart problems, and it wasn't until I ended up in a hospital emergency room that I learned my condition was called Ehlers-Danlos Syndrome and was the precursor of many problems to come. According to the National Ehlers-Danlos Foundation, EDS is fairly uncommon and is thought to affect 1 in approximately 5,000 people worldwide. It is found in both males and females of all racial and ethnic backgrounds. Ehlers-Danlos Syndrome is a group of inherited connective tissue disorders which are characterized by joint hypermobility, skin extensibility, and fragile tissue. People with EDS have a defect in their connective tissue. It's this tissue that provides support to many body parts such as skin, muscles, ligaments, and organs. The fragile skin and unstable joints found in EDS patients are due to faulty collagen. Collagen is a protein that acts like glue in the body, adding strength and elasticity to connective tissue.

There are six types of Ehler-Danlos Syndrome. The type I have is most closely associated with the Classical type, with manifestations of stretchy skin, easy bruising, widened scaring, and joint hypermobility (sprains & dislocations). In my teen years I had several instances of dislocations of my left shoulder. The skin is soft and velvety almost dough like with scaring found mostly over pressure points such as knees, elbows forehead and chin. Muscle tone and delayed gross motor development may also be evident. A particular type of EDS will run true within individual families, as seems to be the case in mine.

My mother had Ehlers-Danlos Syndrome and it was genetically passed on to me. It seems to have run male, female in our family. My mother's father had the condition, his mother had it, her father had it, and so on, as far back as we know. My mother had a brother who did not have the condition and none of his children; a girl and two boys were affected. I have two sisters who do not have the condition and none of their children; five girls and one boy are affected. I have one son, who does not have it either. EDS in our family seems to have run father to daughter, mother to son. If I had had a daughter, most likely she would have been born with Ehlers-Danlos Syndrome and she in turn would most likely have passed it on to a son. With me having a son and no biological daughter, my theory at this point is EDS, in our family, may have come to an end. I have no facts or studies for basing my theory, however, looking back through five generations on my maternal grand-father's side of the family, and being from Leicester, England, seems to support my theory. My son has not had any genetic testing, however before he considers having children, he might want to do so. Having children always posed a big question in my mind, with knowing my experiences as a child and not wanting to pass my condition on to another generation, I struggled with the decision of even having children. So when Mike was born a healthy child and did not have EDS, there was great relief on my part.

My mother struggled her whole life with Ehler-Danlos. As I mentioned, she had the same condition as I have, however her health issues were manifested somewhat differently than mine. Raised on a ranch, she would fall and injure herself in the same manner as me, with the same results. However, as a young girl, she had intestinal and digestive issues that continued through her adult years. With age, osteoporosis became an increasing problem causing extreme pain in her neck, hips, and knees. Pain and disfigurement in her hands presented many challenges when trying to perform the simplest tasks. Mom was under care of an arthritic specialist for years undergoing periodic shots of cortisone in her joints to help with pain management and mobility. She was a trouper, always remaining upbeat and cheerful, not wanting to show just how much discomfort she had to endure. The digestive, intestinal, joint, and arthritic problems I have experienced over the years have been much less troublesome than hers, at least at this point in time.

I believe it was in the fall of 1990 that I began having some strange sensations in my chest. I thought it might have been indigestion or acid reflux. I would feel pressure in my chest, light headed, and sweaty. It would happen occasionally and only for brief periods. I didn't think too much about it due to the fact I felt fine the rest of the time. A year earlier at a checkup with my longtime family physician, Dr. Robert Huntington, I might have expressed some concerns in regards to my heart and was referred to a cardiologist, Dr. Gregory Hopkins. During the initial visit, he listened to my heart and took chest x-rays. Everything at that time seemed to be okay. This was sometime in 1989. So jumping forward again to late summer and fall of 1990, these spells became more frequent. My wife Mary and I were in San Francisco for a dinner and a play early in October and while dining, I began having these earlier mentioned symptoms. Still thinking it was acid indigestion, we stopped at a nearby pharmacy to pick up some antacid. Mary drove us straight home without even seeing the play. By the time we arrived back in Santa Rosa, I felt fine once again. This was on a Thursday evening. The following day I stayed home from work and was able to get an appointment late in the day with Dr. Huntington. He ran an EKG, listened to my heart, and sent me home saying everything appeared to be okay. Early the following morning, Saturday, I was driving Mary to a scheduled school class and passed out on the way. Seeing me slumped over, she yelled, "Don" which must have been enough to bring me out of my trance. I managed to pull the car over to the side of the road where after getting into the driver's seat, she turned the car around and brought me back home. Mary then went on to the class. The original plan was for me to take her to the class, and pick her up later in the afternoon. As the day transpired, another plan of attack might have been smarter. As the morning progressed, the symptoms became more severe than I had ever experienced before, with accelerated heartbeat, pressure in the chest, lightheadedness, and sweating. Knowing I couldn't drive myself to the hospital, I called my mother who in turn called my brother-in-law, Jack, who came directly, taking me to the ER at Santa Rosa Memorial Hospital.

While in the emergency room, I was fortunate enough to be paid a visit from Dr. Hopkins, the cardiologist I had seen the year earlier, who just happened to be on call that day. He immediately got me started on a series of tests, EKG, echocardiogram, and a heart biopsy. The biopsy was performed thinking I might have contracted a virus in my heart. Later that afternoon, Dr. Hopkins came into my room and told me my situation was very serious, that I had an enlarged heart with a leaky mitral valve. The term he used was cardiomyopathy. My heartbeat would become irregular and very fast paced, (tachycardia) to the point of not pumping blood properly. This placed the heart in a very ineffective and compromising position, thus explaining the reason for all my symptoms. Of course, I was scared to death, with the uncertainty of what might lie ahead. I said, "I don't want to die, I am too young for all of this."

I was admitted and was to stay in ICU at the hospital until Monday, when Dr. Hopkins had made arrangements for me to be transported by ambulance to Sequoia Hospital in Redwood City, California, which is just south of San Francisco. I remember the ride in the ambulance with two attendants and a nurse and being all wired up with heart monitoring equipment. It was a strange feeling viewing the world on my back, facing backward, and watching Mary and my mother following behind in our car. It will always be an unforgettable experience. At Sequoia Hospital, they were to perform, what was referred to as electrophysiological studies on my heart. With these, cardiologists would force my heart to perform in a desired manner electrically.

Next, particular drugs would be introduced into my body to see which combinations of those drugs would correct the tachycardia and help the cardiomyopathy. The reason for being transported to Sequoia was Memorial at that time was not performing these studies. After two weeks of testing, the right combination of medications was decided upon and I was able to return home.

Sequoia Hospital was state of the art when it came to heart care. One complete floor of was designated to studies, research, and care of the heart. In fact, Dan Reeves, an all pro football player and coach had been a patient at the hospital a year or so earlier. Hearing that, I felt I was in a good place. During my stay at Sequoia, we learned that one of my doctors had invented the defibrillator a few years earlier. He had previously received a degree in electrical engineering and later earned a medical degree, specializing in cardiology, where he then used his combined fields of knowledge to invent the defibrillator. The early defibrillators were external units and were too large for chest implantation. The units today are much smaller, smaller than maybe the size of an iPod, and implanted in an area in the upper left chest, to the right of the shoulder and just below the collar bone. As with all of our modern day electronics becoming smaller, one can only imagine how much smaller a defibrillator might become in the future. During my stay at Sequoia, there was discussion that I might have been a candidate for a defibrillator at that time, however, that avenue wasn't taken, seeing how well I responded to the new medications.

Defibrillators are implanted when a poorly performing heart has the chance of stopping. The device monitors the heart function and if the heart should stop, the defibrillator shocks the heart back into rhythm until it's beating properly again on its own. These implanted devices offer the same benefit as provided by external paddles that emergency personnel would use to shock a stopped heart back into action.

2
Realization of Don's Illness

Mary

The first time I realized there was something wrong with Don's health was on a Thursday in early October of 1990. I had gotten up early that morning to get my clothes ready for that evening because we were meeting after work to go to a play in San Francisco. We had inherited fantastic seats from Don's parents for the light opera series. They had been improving their seats for years and asked us if we wanted to take them over. I was so excited about the play that night because it was La Cage aux Folles. I had been talking about it a school for weeks. One of the teachers had jokingly told me that he would love to take the tickets off my hands if I really didn't want to go. I rushed around school all day getting my lesson plans prepared for the next day so I could leave as soon as school was finished. I left school, hurried home to change my clothes, and rushed down to Petaluma to pick up Don. We left his work car there and drove one car to San Francisco. Before the play, we were having dinner at Scott's Seafood Restaurant where we started with escargot. Don had taken only a few bites when he said he didn't feel well. I told him it was probably nothing and told him it would probably go away if he ate some more. But it didn't. And before we got to the entree, he said he needed to leave. Don kept telling me he had a sinking feeling in his chest. We got into the car, however we only made it to the next block where we stopped at a Walgreens to get some antacids. He tried them with no success and though he knew it wouldn't be what I wanted to hear, he asked if we could skip the play and go right home.

The next day was Friday. I went to work, where I had to inform my friend that the tickets did not get used the night before. He was very disappointed that they were wasted tickets. Don stayed home to make an appointment to see his family doctor, who he had been seeing for years. He got in to see Dr. Huntington that afternoon and I met him there after school. They ran some tests on him, one of which was an EKG, that I had never seen performed before. Since then, I have seen it done numerous times. After reading the tests, the doctor said everything seemed to be fine and he would send a report to Dr. Hopkins' office.

So we went home and since Don seemed better, plus the doctor's diagnosis said he was doing well, we had a romantic dinner and evening. The next morning I was taking a math class for teachers in Wikiup, not too far north of Santa Rosa. Don offered to drive me there and pick me up in the afternoon. We started down Fountain-grove Parkway, when all of a sudden the car started veering to the left. I screamed, "Don," because his head was leaning against the window and I thought he had passed out. I tried to reach my left foot over to the brake pedal, luckily by then he had popped out of his trance. I convinced him to let me drive back home. He seemed fine but tired. I know now I should have stayed with him, but he said he was fine and I went on to my class. Many times you read about an automobile accident in a newspaper where a car has gone off the road, overturned, and has killed the occupant, leading the reader to wonder what was the contributing factor. Who knows how many times this scenario has played out in the occurrence of automobile accidents. How so very, very fortunate we both were.

In this day and age it is difficult to believe, however I didn't have a cell phone and because it was Saturday, the school office was locked, thus I had no access to a phone. When I finally arrived home late in the afternoon, Don wasn't there, but his car was in the garage. I immediately called his mother who informed me that Don had had another episode and she in turn called Don's brother-in-law, Jack to take him to the emergency room at Memorial Hospital. I don't think I have ever driven so fast in my entire life. I found myself to the entrance to the ER in a matter of minutes. Rushing in, giving them my husband's name, and being ushered to one of the cubicles took another thirty seconds. There I saw Don lying on an examination bed, calmly talking and laughing with Dr. Hopkins. The first thing out of my mouth was, "Oh my gosh, did having wild sex last night do this to him?" Both of them held back their laughs to tell me that Don had a serious heart condition related to his skin issues. I was relieved to hear I hadn't done anything to harm him, but at the same time I was scared he was dying.

They took Don up to ICU where he stayed until Monday morning when the doctors told us they were transferring him to Sequoia Hospital in Redwood City. There they had specialists that were going to run some tests that would hopefully find medication that would regulate his heart to stave off a heart transplant even though the doctors had informed us it probably was inevitably in Don's future.

Don's mother and I drove down every day after I had sent two of our children, Robert and Tara off to school, left lesson plans at school for the substitute, and made arrangements for our children to go somewhere after school until I got home late at night. Sometimes I didn't make it home until well after commute time had passed, just in time to go to bed and do it all over again the next day. Although it was only for two weeks, I was exhausted. The hospital was very kind to me one weekend by allowing me to stay overnight. Unfortunately, the only bed available was in maternity. It was better than driving home, but I listened to babies crying all night long, thus not a lot of sleep. Don did appreciate that I was able to be there early for him the next day. I was so tired that I fell asleep on Don's bed. He walked down to the nurses' station and informed them that there was a strange woman asleep in his bed. They had monitors on each bed which showed me asleep, so they all had a great laugh while I slept beautifully.

3
Meeting New Doctors

Don

I was informed by Dr. Hopkins while in ICU at Memorial Hospital that in all probability someday I would be headed for a heart transplant. However, with a watchful eye, a series of medications, and periodic testing, we would try to extend that time frame out as far as possible, which we understood could be as long as ten years. This was a bad news, good news scenario. With my diagnosis, he also said that I would be seeing him on a regular basis for the rest of my life. I don't think at that time I wanted to believe what he was saying or maybe I was in denial with the prospect of ever needing a heart transplant,

After returning home from Sequoia Hospital, I pretty much returned to my former schedule of working every day and adjusting to my new series of medications. The first couple of months back working, Dr. Hopkins thought it best if I didn't drive until a pattern could be seen as to how well the new medications would control my heart. My mother, who was still driving at that time, would pick me up daily from my house and drive me to the transit mall. I would take the bus to work and she would pick me up from the terminal in the afternoons. Some days Mary would take me and pick me up depending on her school teaching schedule. By the end of 1990, I returned to driving and once again began working in the yard and undertaking projects around the house. I was on a recipe of high power drugs for probably the next couple of years, being monitored every three month with office visits, echocardiograms, and blood work. The idea of using these drugs was not intended for long term treatment due to increased chances of side effects. So after approximately two years, Dr. Hopkins though it best if I had the electro-physiological studies done again with the idea of taking me off the high powered drugs. This time the studies were performed locally at Santa Rosa Memorial Hospital instead of having to drive all the way to Redwood City. The results proved I could be treated effectively and safely with drugs that possessed fewer long term consequences. With the new assortment of drugs, I actually felt better and was re-lieved they were more compatible for long term use. I continued on this program for some time with occasional minor adjustments.

Starting in 1992 and for the next several years my health situation held fairly stable with visiting Dr. Hopkins every three months and echocardiograms twice a year. Echocardiograms are not too un-like sonograms that women experience during pregnancies. Instead of looking at a baby in the womb echocardiograms view the heart. In my case, looking at the size of the heart, the leaky mitral valve, comparing to prior echoes six month before, and seeing if the heart had become larger, and less efficient were all important aspects of tracking my health. The best we could expect was that the size of the heart hadn't increased since six months prior. During this time, we felt very pleased that testing results did show the condition of the heart had stabilized, not really getting much better, but not getting any worse.

My quality of life and daily routines were once again similar to what they were before all the crazy heart stuff began. Work days consisted of driving to and from Petaluma, California, where I worked as vice president of Kresky Signs, Inc., which is a half hour drive south of my home in Santa Rosa. Kresky Signs is a manufacturer and supplier of graphics and signage for the transportation and construction industries as well as government entities. My days were full days, five days a week, eight hours a day. Weekends were always busy with the kids and their activities and projects around our home. I didn't feel my energy level was compromised much during those years. I even started back snow skiing, of course with the approval of Dr. Hopkins. Skiing was something I had participated in during my younger years and felt I was a half way decent skier. Now you might ask, "Skiing? Are you nuts? With your skin condition and now heart problems, aren't you afraid you will fall and tear open you skin, injuring yourself badly? What about the altitude and breathing issues? After all, you have a bad heart and didn't you say you couldn't participate in contact sports?"

It's kind of funny. As I have become older, I have learned to be more aware of taking proper precautions in my daily activities whether I am working in the yard, projects around the house, exercising, or in sporting activities. Simply by being more in tune with my surroundings, I have tried to develop a sense of what is safe for me physically and not subjecting myself to hazardous situations where I might end up with a severe wound. So again you say,

"Skiing!" The thing about skiing is that you have all this protective gear on; big, heavy boots, that come half way up your calf, thermal underwear, thick ski pants, a heavy ski jacket, thick gloves, goggles, and a ski cap. I always felt as though I was clothed in a suit of armor. With all that protection I could be somewhat aggressive and take on the more challenging runs. I never felt this way with baseball or basketball, which really did not offer much in the way of protection. Swimming, of course did not offer any protection, but really all you are dealing with is water.

In all my years of skiing, never did I ever tear open my skin. Sure, I would fall. Every skier falls, however, my suit of armor always provided protection. High altitude is another area of concern for people with congestive heart failure. With skiing at elevations from 7,000 to 9,000 feet, the air is somewhat thinner and is likely to cause breathing problems for someone who has a compromised heart function. Dr. Hopkins said, "Go ahead and try it." If I had issues, I would know if it was necessary to stop. Much to my pleasure, I didn't have any problems and my breathing seemed to be fine. In fact, I felt better in the cold dry air.

In 1998 we purchased a vacation home in the Lake Tahoe area, spending many weekends and vacations with family and friends. Skiing the beautiful trails of the exceptional ski resorts in the winter months and golfing, swimming, fishing, hiking, rafting, or long leisurely walks during the summer months, were all activities I truly cherished. When we had friends up for a skiing weekend, they would have contests with me to see how many ski runs we could get in during the day. Often, 15 - 20 runs from 9:00 to 3:00, with a break for lunch, was considered a successful day. Riding the chair lift up the mountain, I would contemplate my last run of the day. I also anticipated the cold wind at my face and preparing myself mentally for the challenging run with the difficult moguls and somewhat icy conditions. I knew at the bottom of the hill I would be rewarded with an ice cold Sierra Nevada Pale Ale after a day of successfully conquering the ski slopes.

Part of my motivation on a daily basis was to push myself physically, trying to extend my limit further each time with the idea that I could still accomplish everything I used to. Maybe again it was denial, but I felt I had to prove to myself I could still function at a high level. Whether it was climbing stairs at work or at home, mowing the lawn, riding the bicycle, walking the hills in our neighborhood, or working out at the gym, I was always checking to see that my baseline had not declined. If I was headed for a heart transplant, I was going down fighting. Through the 90s and into the early 2000s, I continued to function at a fairly high level. I would become somewhat winded and out of breath participating in the previously mentioned activities, however I continued pushing forward.

It was late 1999 or early in 2000 that I began to have bladder problems. For some years before, the emptying of my bladder had become more and more difficult. I had prostate checks with PSA blood screenings and there were no issues. I has visited Dr. James Palleschi, a well-respected Santa Rosa urologist, for several years and when I complained of increased problems with emptying my bladder, he performed more studies, one of which was a cystoscopy, where a light is inserted through the urethra and into the bladder. It was found that I had an enlarged bladder with an extra part or sac on one side, called a diverticulum. Basically, what I had was two bladders. Over time, my bladder had become weakened and was not able to efficiently eliminate the urine. The cause of this was once again the result of having Ehlers Danlos Syndrome. The walls of the bladder had lost the ability to constrict properly, thus creating issues with eliminating urine in an effective manner. This problem did not allow the urine to be completely drained, and with some urine remaining in the bladder, the bladder became weaker and less effective, with increased chances of developing urinary tract infections. Dr. Palleschi prescribed medications which would help the bladder constrict with better flow of urine. These drugs helped in a limited way. However, he felt I was headed for what was referred to as intermittent self-catheterization, but at the same time he wanted me to visit a colleague of his, Dr. Wendy Leng at UC Medical Center in San Francisco for a second opinion.

In the spring of 2000, we made the drive to San Francisco for the second opinion. All the while driving, I complained of the shit I was having to experience and would these unpleasant medical issues ever cease. Waiting impatiently in the examination room for the doctor to come in, and still having a fit in regards to the procedure I was about to endure, the door opened and my whole demeanor changed when I gazed upon one of the most beautiful female doctors I had ever seen. She asked how I was doing and all I could say was, "Great!" She could have performed almost any procedure or test on me at that moment and I would have loved it. She did perform a cystoscopy and it confirmed what Dr. Palleschi had earlier thought to be the case with my condition. I was shown how to perform self-catheterization with the insertion of a catheter through the urethra and into the bladder, for eliminating my urine. I was to perform this unpleasant procedure as needed several times a day. As I settled in with this experience I found three or four times a day was sufficient, usually morning, midday, and evening. However, the procedure did not come without challenges. Keeping clean and sterile was a constant issue, especially at work and traveling, where there wasn't the comfort or cleanliness of my own bathroom. The avoidance of infection was a constant worry. Even when I felt I had taken all the precautions for being sterile and clean, the introduction of bacteria into the urinary tract was difficult to prevent. Every few months I would get an infection. After taking a urine specimen to the lab, Dr. Palleschi's office would get me started on an antibiotic, usually Cipro. Sometimes other antibiotics were prescribed. After a couple of weeks, I was good to go again for another few months.

I found over time I got used to my new program. After all, what choice did I have? I would have to perform this procedure for the rest of my life because performing intermittent catheterization prevents the bladder's ability for eliminating urine on its own. Doing anything repeatedly and often enough becomes second nature. I became quite adept at performing my newly prescribed routine. Although, that might not be what I would want inscribed on my headstone. Having some levity helps in keeping a sane mind. I also find that being somewhat detached mentally from preforming the procedure allows me to be emotionally better to deal with it. Sometimes it's as though I am seeing someone else in the picture and it's not really me.

Traveling by car or airplane presented some very interesting challenges for my intermittent catheterization process. Whether we were driving by car to the mountains, Palm Desert, or flying to Cancun or Hawaii, you haven't lived until you have tried performing the catheter insertion procedure in the back seat of your car, in a dirty service station bathroom, or at a roadside rest stop. But the best was trying to maneuver my paraphernalia within the confines of a two foot by three foot jetliner restroom at thirty-five thousand feet over the Pacific or Caribbean Oceans.

The beginning of our new decade 2000 offered very few changes in my day to day activities and I continued to remain very active. However, during the fall of 2003, we had made plans with our friends for a Caribbean cruise during Thanksgiving week. The week leading up to our departure I began not feeling well. I thought I might have come down with a virus or a cold. So as a precaution, I made an appointment with my current general practitioner, Dr. Tim Pile, to check me out in hopes of giving me something for whatever was bothering me. I told him we were leaving for Fort Lauderdale for a cruise the following day. He did an EKG and listened to my chest. When he came back into the examination room, he informed me that I was not going on any cruise. My heart was not in any condition for travel. He immediately faxed the results of the EKG over to Dr. Hopkins' office and I was instructed to call for an appointment the following day. But I said, our bags are packed and waiting by the front door and our friends were already in Florida waiting for us. I asked Dr. Pile to call my wife and tell her the bad news. She would never believe me! In fact, she didn't even believe Dr. Pile and thought it was a joke. I remember leaving his office in total bewilderment as to what had just transpired. How could I ruin a trip at the very last minute. To this day, I don't think I will ever live that down. We called our friends and told them the news. It was fortunate I had purchased travel insurance. On the cruise, our friends overheard the couple who at the very last minute got a great deal on our stateroom say, "How would anyone ever give up these wonderful accommodations?" As it turned out, it was a blessing we did not make the trip. I might have had a burial at sea.

Upon having the cardiology appointment with Dr. Hopkins and the usual work-up of echocardiogram, blood testing and listening to my heart, he wanted me to have an angiogram. An angiogram is performed by the insertion of a catheter, usually through the femoral artery and injecting a contrast die which allows by means of x-ray, viewing of the coronary arteries of the heart. The procedure was scheduled at Sutter Medical Center in Santa Rosa where a new angio/cath lab had recently been completed. So while our friends were having a wonderful time cruising the Caribbean, I was having my own vacation at the hands of Dr. Hopkins. The results of the procedure was that I needed a defibrillator implanted into my chest. My first reaction was, I don't want to have one! I thought it was something optional. I guess it was my option. However, Dr. Hopkins said, "Do you want to die?" Well, I guess I am not that stupid. Dr. Hopkins felt the implantation of a defibrillator was a must. I was completely in shock. With my condition evidently not improving, my heart had a chance of just stopping. The implantation of the defibrillator would be an insurance policy. If my heart did stop, the device would shock the heart back into action. After digesting the latest news and knowing there was really no other choice, I said, "We had better do it." This was probably just a stop gap on the way to someday needing a heart transplant. But many people have defibrillators and lead completely normal lives. In fact, I have three friends who have implanted defibrillators and are doing just fine. We would see what lies ahead after receiving the defibrillator.

So we got the surgery scheduled at Santa Rosa Memorial Hospital for some time in December to be performed by Dr. Peter Chang Sing, who specializes in defibrillator implantation. Everything went fine as expected and with an overnight stay for making sure the leads to the heart were in proper position, I was able to return home the following day. For the next three weeks I was to have very limited use of my left arm with no lifting so as to insure the leads didn't become dislodged during the healing process. So by the first part of

January 2004, I was almost as good as new. The only physical evidence of my new piece of equipment was a small scar and a raised area in the skin just below my left collar bone.

Once again, we were back on the right track, back to working full time and even back on the ski slopes. With some adjustments to my medicines, the addition of blood thinners, a constant watchful eye on my diet (low sodium), and every three month visits with Dr. Hopkins, we continued trying to push that heart transplant down the road.

The first part of 2004 was seemingly a good period of time with a full schedule of working, including trips to Palm Desert, and our annual week's visit to Cancun the end of April. However, by spring that year, after another office visit with Dr. Hopkins, and with the usual program of tests, he recommended I see a friend of his, Dr. Michael Fowler at Stanford University Hospital. The two of them had been roommates while attending Stanford Medical School together some years earlier. Dr. Fowler had stayed on at Stanford and was the director of the heart failure program. I thought I was in fairly good health for the shape I was in, but Dr. Hopkins thought it best that I go down to Stanford and at least talk to Dr. Fowler. It was set up for a June visit and so down we went, about a two hour drive. Little did we realize this visit was the first of many for years to come. I am sure Dr. Hopkins knew, what was lying in wait for me.

Of course, I was very nervous and apprehensive in regards to having another doctor and hospital looking into my situation. As you can imagine, by this time I was becoming very sick and tired of my health program. With watching my diet, doctor and hospital visits, lab work, defibrillator checks, bladder and catheter issues, my monitoring of activities, and medicine adjustments, the process almost became a full time job. It was almost as though I didn't have time for anything else. But we trudged forward, never giving up the thought that someday we would be beyond all of this craziness.

Dr. Hopkins had previously sent my records down to Dr. Fowler, so when we met, he would be up to speed with my condition. I remember nervously waiting for my first appointment in the cardiac clinic at Stanford Hospital. It seemed we waited for hours. Of course, it probably seemed longer, with all the new and strange surroundings. There were patients in wheelchairs, some trying to maneuver their walkers, some with oxygen tanks and masks, huffing and puffing as they tried to navigate about the overcrowded waiting rooms. I thought, is this going to be me?

Are these people pre or post-surgery? It was a very unsettling situation! Staff, doctors, and medical students in white coats were hurrying about, tending to their daily duties. The longer I waited, the more anxious I became, with my blood pressure increasing by the minute. Of course, the first thing they do is to weigh you and take your blood pressure. My white coat syndrome by then had really kicked in. I don't recall what my blood pressure was at the time, but knowing how I reacted to stressful situations, I know it was quite high.

Stanford University Hospital is different than many city or regional hospitals due to being a teaching hospital, part of a university, and a major trauma center. Many of the doctors you see, whether it's for heart, kidney, lungs, or whatever the specialty might be, are also in many cases professors at Stanford University Medical School. So the halls of the hospital are full of doctors, medical students, interns, and senior fellows. Add to that, nurses, staff, patients being wheeled about, family members, and other visitors, the atmosphere is very overwhelming for a first time experience.

Meeting Dr. Fowler was a pleasant encounter. He was very accommodating, personable, and friendly. Mary and I both liked him very much. His low keyed, almost comedic approach made for a more relaxed situation, without being cavalier in regards to the importance of the visit. The appointment was pretty much a get-acquainted chat with discussing my background and medical history; Ehlers Danlos Syndrome, bladder, etc.. We talked about the potential of having a heart transplant and that Dr. Norman Shumway performed the first heart transplant in the United States at Stanford University in 1968. Stanford currently performs approximately 50 heart transplants a year and is considered one of the premier facilities for heart care in the United States. Heart transplantation is the last choice in treating patients with congestive heart failure, when all other avenues of treatment have been exhausted. However, in several years with advancements in stem cell research there may be other options available for treatment. After a physical examination and listening to my heart, Dr. Fowler left me on my same program of medications and stressed no salt or alcohol, which I already knew and was abiding by. Although, the occasional meal of dining out was somewhat challenging when it came to no salt. However, I felt I had stayed away from the transplant table by watching my diet and I certainly was not about to ignore that now. We ended our visit by setting up the next appointment for the following month.

On one of our clinic visits with Dr. Fowler, he arranged an appointment for us to meet Mary Burge, a pre-heart transplant coordinator and a social worker who evaluated our suitability for a heart transplant. Dr. Fowler, knowing what I was most likely headed for, thought it best to get the ball rolling by checking my background, family history, and support group. Her job was to prepare us and teach us about a heart transplant. She showed us a video and provided us with a packet of information for study at home. All of this information was extremely beneficial to us in learning what was involved and answered many questions.

We were approaching fall, and on one of our visits with Dr. Fowler, he talked about the possibility of my having a heart valve repair. He felt performing a valve repair might help the leaky mitral valve function more efficiently. The leaky valve and cardiomyopathy (enlarged heart) were two of the underlying factors of my condition. A valve repair, would hopefully, provide for better pumping of blood throughout my body, instead of leaking back into the heart. With a compromised heart function, a person's body does not receive the proper blood supply and oxygen needed in helping the body's tissues and organs efficiently perform their designed tasks. We were informed by Dr. Fowler my condition was like being on a slippery slope. One day I would be okay and feeling fine and possibly the next day, the next week, or the next month, I might not be feeling or functioning as well. So it was very important to remain proactive in the approach to my care and treatment.

So at the end of September 2004, we had an appointment with Dr. Philip Oyer, a cardiothoracic surgeon at Stanford who served his internship and residency at Stanford School of Medicine and Stanford University Hospital in the 1970s. He was currently associate chair at the school of medicine. His office was in a large building adjacent to the hospital. We took an elevator up to the second floor which opened up to an enormous room filled with many office cubicles, most being occupied by staff working on computers at desks. I thought maybe we had made a wrong turn and ended up at an investment brokerage firm or the headquarters of a Silicon Valley hi-tech company. The end of the room held a large conference room and the far wall was lined with office suites, one of which we were ushered into by a staff assistant. There we waited for our meeting with Dr. Oyer. His office was richly appointed with a large desk, bookcases, and plush seating. Once again, it didn't seem like a medical setting. Not having the clinical feeling was probably much better and less intimidating. After a short wait, Dr. Oyer came into the office. We were surprised! I don't know what we were expecting. However, what does a world class heart surgeon supposed to look like anyway? He was probably in his 50s, average height, with a full head of greying hair, mustache, goatee, casual clothes and boots. We had heard sometime earlier he rode motorcycles, so that explained the boots.

Once again, going through all the pleasantries of a first time meeting and while Dr. Oyer was reviewing my case on the computer, he said, "I see your birthday is October 31st. That's mine as well." I knew then this was to be the beginning of a good doctor/patient relationship. He showed pictures of my enlarged, leaky heart in bright living color on his computer, which did not mean much to our eyes, however they were fascinating. Dr. Oyer stated, after studying my case and talking with Dr. Fowler, he felt I would be a candidate for the mitral valve repair. He then showed us a round black plastic or hard rubber part with holes on the outer circumference. It looked as though it could have been a gasket that you would buy at your local auto parts store.

The part had a bar code attached. Of course, we asked what that was about and Dr. Oyer informed us the bar code enables the hospital to know how much to charge. This was meant to be a joke.

Dr. Oyer went over what was involved with the surgery. It would be an open heart surgery, placing the new part into the mitral valve, with the idea of minimizing the leakage of blood back into the heart, thus enabling the heart to be more effective for pumping blood throughout my body. The surgery was to be a three to four hour process, with possibly a week to ten day stay in the hospital for recovery, then returning home, hopefully almost new. Dr. Oyer was to have my surgery scheduled within the following two weeks and we would be notified by his staff assistant when we should return to Stanford Hospital for preparation before surgery.

So we received the call and down we went, sometime before the middle of October. We arrived the day before the surgery for an office visit, lab work, chest x-rays, CT scan, and echocardiogram. With all our previous visits to Stanford, I constantly fought within myself concerning what I was having to experience, instead of embracing the fact that I was being helped toward leading a better life. The thought of a major heart surgery scared me to death.

After the day's pre-op appointments were complete we checked into the SLAC House for lodging that evening. The SLAC House is a guest facility for people visiting Stanford University and is adjacent to the Stanford Linear Accelerator, which is the world's largest and most powerful linear particle accelerator. The device is operated by Stanford University and uses electricity to accelerate and collide subatomic particles. Sorry for the sidebar. Even though we were not members of the scientific community, we qualified because of my special heart. The guest house was fairly new and had rooms which were very small, kind of like college dorm rooms, however very clean. So after checking in, we went out to a local restaurant to enjoy our final meal before surgery and nervously waited for my big day.

We checked in at admitting very early in the morning going directly to pre-op where I was instructed to put on one of those lovely open back hospital gowns. I was then ushered to my bed, which was in a curtained cubicle where I waited for a series of pre-op procedures to take place. With all the activity happening around me and with other patients waiting for surgeries, I didn't have much chance to worry about the cold steel scalpel and power saw that was about to slice open my chest and the trained hands of Dr. Oyer delving into my chest cavity, hoping to repair the leaky valve of my enlarged heart. An IV was placed into a vein of one arm, my chest was shaved, and a blood pressure cuff was secured on my other arm. After discussing my history with nurses and conferring with an anesthesiologist, I was asked to sign some forms. (Sometime previously in preparation for my upcoming surgery, Mary and I had filled out health care directives giving each other power of attorney for health care decisions. In case something would have happened to me during surgery, Mary would have the authority to act as my agent.) Next, I was transported to surgery. Mary followed along beside me until we reached the surgery room doors, leaving me with the thought, "Think sex and I love you," which were always her parting words.

I woke up! I made it! I was alive! I came out from under the anesthesia about the same time the nurses were extracting the endotracheal tube from my throat, which was used for my breathing during surgery. It felt as though they were removing something about the size of a small minivan, when in fact the tube was only about an inch in diameter. Mary informed me that Dr. Oyer had already visited with her in the family waiting room and reported to her that I had come through the surgery with flying colors. He felt the valve repair was just what I needed and thought the procedure would help to improve my situation. He also stated that even with my Ehlers Danlos Syndrome, and with the enlarged inefficient heart, my heart tissue was not too unlike someone's tissue with a so-called normal heart. The other good news was that he didn't have to use the artificial valve. He was able to repair my existing mitral valve. So the part we saw in his office could now be returned to the auto parts store.

I remained in ICU for several days, being closely watched with a heart monitor attached to my chest, and IV drip in my arm, and a blood pressure cuff on the other arm. The catheter had been inserted into my bladder prior to surgery and was to remain there until I was released to go home. I was certainly not in any position for performing the intermittent self-catheterization process on my own, since I had become best friends with a pillow, which I constantly used for holding against my chest every time I coughed or moved. The doctors and nurses expressed the importance of the pillow thing for the protection of my incision. I don't think incision is the proper term. When you have your sternum sawed in half and your chest plate pulled apart, somehow incision sounds too insignificant.

The day I was being transferred from ICU to a regular cardiac room, I glanced over to the person who was in the bed next to me. I had not seen the person prior to being moved because of the curtaining between our two areas. However, I had heard the constant sounds of hissing air and whirling equipment. I remember thinking to myself, "What is going on over there?" Mary had previously mentioned to me on some of her visits about the poor old man in the next bed, and what sad shape he was in. To make matters worse, he never seemed to have any family members who came to visit. I didn't think much in regards to his situation until I was actually wheeled past his cubicle. What I saw, almost scared me into cardiac arrest. He was lying there, mostly naked and unconscious, with hoses, wiring, and tubing coming out of his chest, all of which were attached to various pieces of equipment. He looked to be a man in his late seventies. He had that grey, ashen look you would associate with death. What came to mind was a body in preparation for transition to another world, as if in some science fiction movie. I thought, "Has this man already had a heart transplant or was he waiting for one?" Whatever the case, he was not at all in good shape. We later heard from some of the nursing staff the man was waiting for a new heart and that he was only thirty-seven years old. He was attached to what is referred to as an LVAD, a left ventricle assist device, which mechanically and electrically keeps the heart pumping. Without the device, he most likely would have been dead. All I could think of, in a selfish way, was hoping that that man's condition, heaven forbid, was not going to be me someday. Still to this day, the image of that man constantly haunts me. We never did hear if he received a new heart. We can only hope that he did.

I continued my recovery in the cardiac wing of the hospital for approximately another seven days. Family and friends visited often. My brother-law from Wisconsin, Ed Meyer, had previously sent me a pair of his silk pajamas and robe. Knowing how well they worked for him on one of his hospital visits, he thought they would be just the ticket for me while walking the halls. There is nothing worse that wearing one of those hospital gowns with your butt hanging out the back while pulling along your IV and catheter bag during a walk. My instructions were to walk the halls several times a day. Initially, I was quite weak and unstable, however the more I walked, the stronger I became. Of course, wearing my new outfit gave me more incentive to walk. All I needed was an ascot and a pipe and I could have been Hugh Heffner. There was only one problem. I didn't have a bevy of beautiful women surrounding me. The doctors and nurses continually commented how debonair I looked in my silk Armani outfit. Actually, they were very practical for getting in and out of the hospital bed, instead of those cotton things that became all bound and twisted. I liked my borrowed outfit so much, Mary went over to Macy's at the Stanford Mall and bought me one of my own.

After several more days, we were able to return home. I had to remain in close contact with my pillow whenever I got in or out of bed. When I coughed, it felt like my chest was going to split apart, so holding the pillow against my chest really helped in making me more secure and comfortable. I was not to lift anything with my arms and of course no driving for several weeks. Negotiating stairs was also out of the picture. This presented a problem for me since we live in a two story house. I had to live on our bottom level for the first week, which was okay, since I was still not very sure footed. Somehow, falling down a flight of stairs did not sound very appealing.

After a few weeks, I returned to work. I was still not able to drive and the prospect of getting behind the wheel was daunting to me since my chest was not completely healed as yet. Each day I rode to work with Steve and Audrey. They worked at Kresky with me and lived in Santa Rosa. Mary would drop me off at their house each morning on her way to school and picked me up each evening. This routine continued for a couple of weeks until I could return to driving.

4
Introduction to Stanford Hospital

Mary

O n a beautiful day in March or April of 2000, Don's life was about to take another turn that would change our lives forever. We had been sent down to UCSF to see a urologist. Don was not happy in the least about the prospect of being catheterized for the rest of his life. So on the way driving down to San Francisco and the whole time waiting to be called into the examination room, Don ranted and raved about how he hated being sick all the time and was tired of hospitals and doctors. We got called into the examination room where he continued with his grumbling until the door opened and the most beautiful doctor we had ever seen walked in saying, "Hello, how are you doing Mr. Coover?" Then in the sweetest voice Don replied, "I'm just great doctor, how are you?" I guess I'm mcant to bc Don's sounding board for the tough times. We still have laughs about his change of attitude that day.

The next time that I had to confront the negative aspects of Don's health issues was Thanksgiving week of 2003. We had been planning a Caribbean cruise with six of our friends for about nine months. I had worked hours and hours lining up a substitute and getting lesson plans ready. I was so psyched for this very first cruise of my life. We had bought a ton of new clothes for the formal dinners and I had tried losing weight to look half way decent in a swimsuit. Plus, I had been nonstop talking about the cruise with my friends and co-workers. The suitcases were literally packed and sitting by the front door. We were all set to leave early the next morning. However, as a precaution since he hadn't been feeling well, Don decided to see his current family doctor. When I say my world collapsed that evening, I am not exaggerating. Dr. Pile called at 5:30 pm to say we would not be going on any cruise. At first, I thought he was playing one of his practical jokes, but as the conversation advanced, I knew this was no joke. I am not ashamed to say I cried myself to sleep that night. I know it sounds selfish and you are right. However, all I could do at that time was to feel sorry for myself. Looking back, I can laugh at it all because it turned out to be just the first of other cancelled trips. Now we are old hands at packing and unpacking quickly.

Because of this recent set-back with Don's health, Dr. Hopkins wanted Don to have an angiogram at Sutter Hospital. So we drove over early one morning and after prepping him they took him into the cath lab while I paced back and forth in the waiting room. Don's sister Candi joined me. I was so thankful that she was there when Dr. Hopkins came out to talk to me. He told us that Don should have a defibrillator put in, but he was very clear that this was only a temporary fix. He sat down in front of us in the small, cramped waiting room and calmly said that Don was probably and most likely headed for a transplant down the road. This was a shock for me. I just never thought it was that serious. Although, the possibility of a transplant had been discussed previously, I didn't believe it would actually happen.

Then in December of 2003 we met Dr. Peter Chang Sing who was going to perform the implantation of the defibrillator. We liked him right away. A no nonsense kind of doctor, who explained everything thoroughly to us and answered all of our questions. He had a great bedside manner. We found out much later that he lived just down the street from us. Don had the procedure done at Memorial Hospital which was an overnight stay. However, it's always a huge process every time he goes to the hospital because he has to be catheterized. Most times this ends up meaning he developed a bladder infection, something else having to deal with. While he was at Memorial, there was a gentleman in the bed across from Don who had a defibrillator implanted a few months before. He was back in the hospital for a repair. It seems he had tried to lift a fireplace insert by himself at his home and burst the stitches around the implant. I am sure it was a lesson well learned. Don didn't have a great stay that time because of the moaning patient next to him, but luckily it was just one night. Plus, the doctors and nurses were so attentive that there was little to complain about.

Eventually, Dr. Hopkins felt Don's health had gotten to a point where he needed to see a specialist who dealt with heart transplants. We were sent down to a friend of his, Dr. Fowler, at Stanford Hospital in Palo Alto. Our first time visit was worse than horrible. I bet we sat in the waiting room for at least three hours. During that time Don was a nervous wreck. We don't know if it was just that particular day, but the room was filled to capacity and overflow people were standing and sitting on the floor. Later the hospital sent us a questionnaire about our visit. This in turn must have influenced them to move their offices upstairs for more room. We fell in love with Dr. Fowler at first sight. It was a little overwhelming though, because he talked a mile a minute. He was upbeat and gave you the feeling he genuinely cared about each and every one of his patients. Later on, Dr. Fowler sent us to see Mary Burge, a heart transplant coordinator. I couldn't believe all the questions she asked about our family habits, where we lived and worked, our friends, economic background, insurance plans, plus Don's health history. We know now all that information plays an important role in who is eligible for a transplant. Definitely the people who have a strong family support group are going to have an easier adjustment to a transplant and the following care that is required.

The next doctor we met was Dr. Oyer, a heart transplant surgeon, also from Stanford. Although his appearance was not what we expected, he was funny, light hearted, yet extremely qualified so we were put at ease immediately. Both Don and I loved his sense of humor which was apparent the very first time we met in his office. He put us completely at ease and was most reassuring that this was the right avenue for us to take at this time.

In early October 2004, Dr. Oyer performed the valve repair on Don, who ended up staying at Stanford for two weeks of recovery. Staying at the SLAC House was perfect for me at that time because I really didn't spend a lot of time there. I usually left for the hospital at about 7:00 am and returned after Don had been served his dinner. It was only seventy-five dollars a night and for five dollars a day more I rented a microwave/refrigerator so I could fix a quick breakfast or a cup of soup and some fruit for dinner. I wouldn't recommend it for a long stay, but it was perfect for the two weeks. I had brought some school work down with me and there was a table and television downstairs where I could work. One day some gentlemen came down to watch a football game, saw me with piles of construction paper and scissors, and were about to turn around and leave. I begged them to stay so I could have some company if only for a short while. I think I even watched the game with them which was a shocker for me.

I stayed with Don all day every day mostly knitting or reading books when he slept. Thus, I was very pleased when his two sisters and mother drove down one day to visit. His mother was not feeling well so they borrowed a wheelchair from the lobby of the hospital to wheel her to the second floor to see Don. There wasn't much room by the two beds, so they left the wheelchair in the hallway. When they went to retrieve it, it wasn't there. We all panicked thinking we would have to explain why we couldn't return it to the lobby. It turned out someone had returned it for us thinking we were finished using it. I really did appreciate their visit and was sad to see them leave. Sometimes it was lonely when Don was asleep and I had no one to talk to.

About this same time there seemed to be a strange unpleasant odor coming from Don's room every time I went to visit him. Every day it got worse and worse. Pretty soon I told the nurses I couldn't stand the smell any longer. They gave me some packets that had been warmed up in the microwave with wet cloths in them to bathe him. Believe me, I scrubbed and scrubbed until his skin was red, however the odor persisted. Finally one day I said I couldn't stand it any longer and a nice nurse helped him take a shower. Don was like a new man when he stepped out. And better than that, the whole room no longer had that gagging aroma. We take all those little things like a shower for granted, however it surely lifted my spirits.

5

Defibrillator
& Low-Sodium Diet

Don

By the time we approached the latter part of 2004, my routine was once again not unlike what I had experienced over the prior several years. My activity level was back on par, not too unlike it had been previously, with working every day, projects around the house, and trips to our place in the mountains. However, I had discontinued skiing. I was sixty years old now and did not want to risk a chance of injury. It was a hard decision, but I knew it was the best decision considering all my health issues. We made it through the holidays that year, as I continued with my check-ups at Stanford and with Dr. Hopkins in Santa Rosa. Laboratory blood work, echocardiograms, monitoring the implanted defibrillator, listening to my heart, and adjustments to my prescription regimen remained a part of the ongoing program.

The defibrillator is really a remarkable device. Besides having the ability for shocking a heart that has stopped and pacing it back into rhythm, the defibrillator acts as a computer, constantly recording every beat. So, during an office visit, the technician would place a device over my heart. It almost had the appearance of a computer mouse which was attached to a monitor and a computer. This device electronically extracted all the stored information from the defibrillator that had been produced 24/7 since my last office visit. This information, along with the results of the echocardiogram, would give doctors an update on my heart function and compared that information to previous results.

Results from the echocardiogram, which uses sound waves to produce images of the heart, provides a vast amount of information on the condition and function of that heart. However, with my limited knowledge of what was going on, a term that always had an impact on me, was ejection fraction. Ejection fraction (EF) is a number represented as a percentage on how well or how efficient a heart is performing with pumping blood throughout the body. This is usually measured in the left ventricle, the heart's main pumping chamber. A healthy heart would have an ejection fraction of 50% to 75%. A below normal reading would be 36% to 49%, and a low reading would be under 35%. Well, my (EF) was usually between 22% and 27%, which was not good. A good analogy here would be a low FICO score in measuring someone's financial picture. A FICO score of 500 would be about the same as my 20 something ejection fraction. A 500 FICO score would represent a pretty bleak financial outlook for someone. In the same manner, my low heart performance was giving me a bleak picture of my continued health.

On one of our clinic visits at Stanford with Dr. Fowler, we met a man and his wife who had written no-salt cookbooks. He was also a patient of Dr. Fowler. His name was Donald Gazzaniga. We learned he had been in the Marines and had written the book, "A Few Good Men: The Marines." Some years earlier he had developed congestive heart failure and was headed for the heart transplant list. So he developed many very low sodium, but tasty recipes. Never consuming more than 500 milligrams of sodium a day, with plenty of exercise, and closely watching his medicines, his condition improved dramatically. His improvement has kept him off the transplant list and seeing how well he had improved with a very low sodium diet, we decided to buy his "No-Salt, Lowest Sodium Cookbook, " which became my bible for the next couple of years. Dr. Fowler had written the forward for the book. Since his first low sodium cookbook, he has co-authored several other low sodium cookbooks with his wife and daughter.

With trying many of his recipes, it was really quite amazing just how good foods tasted without the use of salt. Using fresh fruits and vegetables and staying away from canned or packaged foods made it much easier to stay around 500 milligrams of sodium per day. The use of fresh herbs and spices certainly made up for what was lost without using salt. I had been watching my sodium intake for the past several years, but with thanks to Mr. Gazzaniga and his "No-Salt, Lowest Sodium Cookbook," I was able to bring my sodium down to an even lower level.

An example of one of my daily menus follows:

Breakfast

1 serving of shredded wheat cereal—0 mg. of sodium
(sometimes for a change, 1 serving of hot cream of
      wheat cereal)—0 mg.
½ cup of fat free milk—65 mg
8 oz. cranberry grape juice—80 mg
1 slice of low sodium toast,—35 mg
5 sprays. Can't Believe It's Not Butter—15 mg*"
      (original spray type)
Once in a while, as an exchange, I have a cooked egg—65 mg "

Having jam on the low sodium toast helps with improving the flavor, 0 mg. of sodium.

When having the egg, the milk would be eliminated by not having the cereal, so the total sodium for most mornings would be as low as 195 milligrams.

Periodically, as another option, we would make beer bread, instead of using the health store type. Using the spray type of butter, and 0 sodium baking powder, which we found on the internet, the only sodium in the whole recipe would be 18 milligrams in the 12 oz. bottle of beer and 15 milligrams for the spray butter. No salt or egg was added to the recipe, just flour and sugar. The best low sodium baking powder is from Ener-G. You can find it at some health food stores but always at either www.healthyheartmarket.com or help for locating such products is available at www.megaheart.com/wheretobuy.html

Lunch

1 tuna sandwich (no salt added or unsalted packed
        in water type) 2 oz—35 mg.
2 pieces of low sodium bread—70 mg.
1 tsp. mayonnaise —38 mg.
8 oz. can of Sprite—45 mg.
1 apple—0 mg

Total — 188 mg.

Some days I would substitute 3 oz. of fresh non-deli turkey breast (54 mg.) instead of the tuna, which would increase the sodium intake for lunch by 16 milligrams. As another change, some days I would have flavored water (0 mg.) instead of the Sprite. With eliminating Sprite I, could lower my sodium to 143 mg.

Dinner

3 oz. Grilled or barbequed salmon—63 mg.
1 medium baked potato with pepper—36 mg.
& spray butter
½ cup steamed broccoli—12 mg.
Fresh garden salad - lettuce, mushrooms, carrots, tomatoes,
        oil & vinegar dressing,—27 mg.
1 cup green tea—0 mg.
Sometimes, popcorn with spray butter for dessert—15 mg.

Total — 153 mg.

Using the 195 mg. total of sodium for breakfast, sodium intake with my example for one day is 536 milligrams. You might think, that's very boring. Does he eat the same menu every day? No! We would change it up almost every day, with the use of fresh meats, fish, vegetables and fruits that contained similar amounts of sodium, as in my example above. Often, we would have other types of fresh fish; red snapper, or sword fish, a hamburger patty, or chicken breast. Other fresh vegetable choices would be asparagus, green beans, zucchini, or artichokes. Occasionally, we would make pasta with pesto, using fresh basil, walnuts, olive oil, pepper, and two tablespoons of Parmigiano Reggiano cheese. The only sodium in the whole recipe was the cheese, @ 60. mg. It always tasted great and who would know there was no salt? So we felt I had a varied diet, with many choices of foods, and yet always keeping in mind the no salt, low sodium idea. Going forward, we aspired to keep my total sodium intake between 500 – 600 milligrams a day.

The consumption of sodium is something as a public we should be more aware of. I hear people say all the time, " I watch my salt intake," or " I don't cook with or add salt to my food." But that is only a small part in the consumption of sodium. People will ask, "What is sodium?" I don't think the majority of our society makes the connection with salt and sodium. Salt is made up of sodium and we consume more on a daily basis than most of us ever realize. Just look at the labeling on packaged foods. If you were to add up your total intake of daily sodium, you would be shocked. Studies show we should limit our sodium intake to no more than 2300 milligrams per day. Well, if we eat out or consume packaged and processed foods, that total could easily become doubled. Sodium is in almost everything we eat or drink. Take a can of soup and look at the label. There are six hundred to nine hundred milligrams per serving and there are two servings per can. What if you ate the whole can? You would have used up two thirds of your daily allotment with just that one item. An interesting project would be to study the sodium content of all the foods you eat for one day; bread, milk, cereal, cheese, butter, meats, and the list can go on and on. Total the sodium on the packaging and at the end of the day I am sure you will be totally surprised. Besides canned soup, there are thousands of canned or packaged foods where we can all get into big trouble. Just read the packaging! In processed foods, the sodium is there for preservation of the item and for taste. Sometime look at the labeling on a package of frozen pizza. After consuming one of those, you might want to pay a visit to your local cardiologist. People who make a regular diet of fast foods and eating out often can place their health in a dangerous situation. We as a society should do the right thing for our bodies by preparing more home cooked meals with fresh ingredients such as fruits and vegetables. As a public, it is imperative to pass on good eating habits to our children. Of course, with our fast paced lifestyles, something packaged and or pre-made is certainly much easier, however at what price do we pay later? Something to think about, (if it comes from a plant, it's good; if it's made in a plant, watch out.)

Now, the question might be asked, what really does too much salt or sodium do? The body needs a certain amount of sodium to hold water in the blood vessels. If there is too much sodium in a diet, more water will be held in the body, thus the amount of blood increases, making the heart work harder with the chance of causing high blood pressure. High blood pressure, if not controlled, can lead to a heart attack, stroke, and /or kidney disease. So the best chance for avoiding problems is watching your sodium intake. I certainly don't want to sound like I am trying to be clinical here because I don't have the background to do so. Also, I don't want to appear that I know all about blood pressure and sodium. However, with all that I have been through, I have learned some simple adjustments to diet and lifestyle that hopefully will keep me on the right course for years to come.

Even though I had been diligently watching my diet and exercise, my congestive heart failure continued to worsen. I had been feeling well for a few months since the valve repair, but my condition began to change during the early winter months of 2005. My energy level had declined and my breathing had become more sensitive. Walking, climbing stairs, and projects that required some degree of effort became more difficult to perform. I had lost the spring in my step that I had regained after the valve repair. The results of one of my office visits to Dr. Hopkins revealed the valve repair had not proved to be much of a long term fix. My leaky, enlarged heart, once again seemed to be headed in a downward spiral. Was my Ehlers Danlos Syndrome the culprit for not having the tissue strength to support the valve repair or was it just the natural process of a deteriorating heart? I will never know the answer.

Dr. Hopkins referred me to a Dr. Lee, who was a part of Dr. Hopkins' cardiology group. The idea was to have the placement of a third lead from the implanted defibrillator to the left side of my heart. The thought behind this procedure was to hopefully create some electrical stimulation, which would help the weakened heart perform better. We had a couple of appointments with Dr. Lee for assessing my situation and discussing what was involved with the procedure. I referred to it as a procedure, but really, it was another surgery. From the beginning of our appointments, I could tell, Dr. Lee was not very keen on wanting to perform this third lead course of action. He said, "It was just a Band-Aid." I think he felt we were only buying a little time, and it would not really help for long term.

At this point, we were on our last legs of trying to prolong the inevitable; the transplant!

Back to the hospital we went. This time to Sutter Medical Center in Santa Rosa. As I was wheeled into the surgery room, the lady from Medtronic happened to be there. I had met her a year or so earlier, when I received the defibrillator. Medtronic was the manufacturer of the device. The anesthesiologist, Dr. Mundel, whose wife worked with Mary at Steele Lane School, was also in attendance, as well as a couple of nurses. It seemed like we had a party while waiting for Dr. Lee's arrival. The interaction with our little group made for a less stressful situation. While waiting for Dr. Lee, I was informed the defibrillator, which I currently had in my chest, was to be exchanged for a new one with the capability of accommodating the third lead. I thought, during some of our earlier discussions, the third lead would just be attached from the existing device to the heart. That wasn't to be the case. As surgeries go, this was to be rather simple. The new defibrillator, although somewhat larger, was placed in the same position where the old unit had been. The leads were attached and that was it.

I remained in the hospital overnight, again making sure the leads remained in proper placement. After a chest x-ray and a computer check on the device, I was able to return home the following day. As with the original defibrillator installation, I was to limit my activities and no lifting with the left arm for several weeks.

It was the spring months of 2005. Was I as good as new again? I don't know . Probably not! However, I felt as though I had more energy. How long would it last? The third lead course of action seemed to be working for now. On one of my visits to Dr. Hopkins' office, and as he saw me walk in, he said, "You have spring in your step." I stated that once again I felt much better. I reported to him that I even negotiated his twenty something steps from the building's entrance up to his office in an aggressive manner. During the previous visit to the building, I had to take the elevator. He seemed to be impressed. The results of the echocardiogram showed that there had been some improvement in my ejection fraction. Not significant, but at least an improvement. I was to remain on the same course of action as I had been following; low sodium and no alcohol. I mentioned to Dr. Hopkins that we had been using " The No-Salt, Lowest Sodium Cookbook," which was an excellent source for reducing my sodium intake. The periodical blood work-ups and the monitoring of blood thinners was to continue. The heart and blood pressure medicines continued in allowing my heart to function with as little stress as possible. Keeping my blood pressure and heart rate at a low level was extremely important.

Surprisingly, for the next several months, it was like old times. Going to the exercise club for light workouts, riding the stationary bike, walking on the treadmill, and using light weights was a frequent routine. I felt re-charged. I could once again mow the lawns and work in the yard. Climbing stairs in our house wasn't as challenging as had been the situation some months earlier. We went to our place in the Tahoe area several times during the summer. I was concerned the altitude might have been an issue. I felt even better in the altitude. If I didn't know differently, I would have thought, "What heart condition?" During this period, my mother's health situation began declining and problems developed at my work which required my attention. I was in a position to approach these issues with the proper attitude because of my renewed physical condition. This allowed me to be in a better place mentally for handling these challenges.

Some months earlier we had traded our timeshare week in Cancun for a week in St Martin. We had the trip scheduled for June, 2005 after Mary had finished teaching for the year. However, after the issue with a new defibrillator and the third lead, we thought it best not to take a trip to foreign country where if I did have a problem and not having the availability of good heart care, we might be subjecting to a potentially dangerous situation. So we asked our son Rob if he and his wife Jennifer if they would be interested in using our week. They jumped at the chance to be able to go. The two of them had a wonderful time experiencing the French and Dutch cultures the island had to offer. And when we learned they came back from their vacation pregnant, of course, Mary and I took some credit. Rob and Jennifer had been trying for some time. So by providing them with the perfect venue, naturally we claimed our share of their success.

My mother, who had lived alone and had taken care of herself for seventeen years since my father had passed away in December of 1988, started developing some health issues. Trips to the doctor's office for an infected leg and arthritis were frequent occurrences as well as a hospital stay for the installation of a pacemaker. I remember talking in the hospital with the cardiologist that performed the pacemaker procedure on Mom and he telling us the tissues of her heart were the consistency of trying to stitch butter. Her advanced years and Ehlers-Danlos had taken their toll. We could see her becoming weaker and failing rapidly. Family members took turns staying with her at night. We continued this program for maybe a month or two until one evening, sometime after the middle of August, we took her to the emergency room at Santa Rosa Memorial Hospital. She been suffering from severe abdominal pains that particular day. The pains seemed different and much more severe than the frequent issues that had plagued her since childhood. Mom had endured pain much of her life in dealing with the arthritis and intestinal problems, so when she said she wanted to be taken to the hospital, we knew we had to act quickly. All these issues were a part of our inherited Ehlers-Danlos Syndrome. Mom passed away from a perforated duodenum on September 1, 2005, just two months shy of her 88th birthday.

Mom always felt badly knowing she had passed the EDS on to me. However, as I said earlier, there wasn't a name attached to the condition when I was born. The condition was just thought to be a hyper-elastic skin. There was never any idea of manifestations into more serious health issues. I felt relieved Mom did not have to witness and be a part of what was lying ahead for me. I can't imagine there could be anything much worse than seeing a son or daughter struggle through severe health problems and not being able to do anything about it.

My sisters and I tended to the sale of Mom's house and getting her estate distributed. We had everything mostly wrapped up by the end of the year. I remember through the listing process, loading our power lawn mower into the back of our SUV and taking it down to Mom's house for mowing her lawn. I must have performed this process several times with no issues. I was actually quite amazed I could lift the mower in and out of the vehicle besides mow and trim both rear and front lawns. I huffed and puffed a little, however, I was thrilled I could accomplish something fairly physical with no ill effects. The bandage was still working!

I celebrated my sixty-first birthday that year on October 31, 2005. Mary had a surprise birthday party for me with family and friends. It had been fifteen years since the heart situation had developed. But with excellent care I had been receiving and proper diet, (low sodium), I was still hanging in there. During all these years though, I constantly looked in the obituaries on a daily basis to make sure my name was not listed.

We made it through the holidays that year. We even took a trip to Palm Desert for Thanksgiving. And Christmas was as great as always with our children and grandchildren. However, by the first of the new year, once again I began not feeling well. That slippery slope had reared its ugly head again. I guess that Band-Aid was now only hanging on by a thread. I felt cold most of the time. The color of my skin was grey and yellow. People would look at me and knew immediately I was not well. Our friends Jim and Donna and John and Janet came over on Super Bowl Sunday to watch the game. Seeing how badly I looked, they only stayed for a short time. My breathing became more labored. Walking up our stairs became more challenging. The results of an office visit to Dr. Hopkins confirmed my heart condition was not headed in a positive direction. The ejection fraction had become worse since it was last checked and the defibrillator monitoring showed my heart had had several PVCs (Premature Ventricular Contractions), which are fairly common in cardiomyopathy patients. The PVCs were mostly unnoticed by me unless I checked my pulse. Only then could I detect the hesitations or irregular beats. Blood screenings and a watchful eye on my medications remained the course of action.

Through all of this, I carried on working every day. I would bundle up in warm clothing, always wearing a hat with the hope of efficiently using the little heat my body produced. I reflect back today on that period of time and wonder how I continued to work. I guess my fighting spirit wouldn't let me give in. I don't feel it was a denial issue. By this time I was fully in acceptance of what was lying in wait.

I remember Mary making a delicious lobster tail Valentine's dinner for me on February 14, 2006. The two of us were sitting at a card table Mary had set up right in front of the living room fireplace. I was all bundled up trying to stay warm. I tried enjoying the meal, however my appetite was just not there. All I could think of was going upstairs and lying down in bed. This increasingly had become my new routine. Even though I went to my work during the day, by evening I was whipped. The process of climbing the nineteen steps, from our living room up to the bedroom, was quite an event. I would have to stop a couple of times to catch my breath before proceeding.

I would never want to experience again those months of February, March, and April. That time frame involved several trips to Memorial Hospital's emergency room. Most of them were evening or late night visits. I would retire to our bedroom early most evenings, but not able to fall asleep. I would lay there in the dark, coughing and listening to my irregular heart beat and worrying if I would wake up in the morning. On some of these occasions, I would wake Mary, telling her I did not feel well. We would get ourselves to the emergency room where doctors would listen to my chest and review my medical history. After a few hours, we were sent home saying there was not much more that could be done. However, on one of these visits a blood test was performed, called a B-type Natriuretic Peptide (BNP) blood test, which measures the level of BNP in a person's blood, indicating the degree of heart failure. The level of BNP below 100 pg/ml indicates no heart failure. The scale of BNP increases through various degrees all the way up to a reading of 900 BNP and above. If I am remembering correctly, my reading was at 900, which denotes severe heart failure. I always knew early on with my original diagnosis that I had congestive heart failure (CHF). I just never remembered seeing a number attached to it. Although the way I currently felt, I knew I was in pretty dire straits.

During one of my emergency room visits, Dr. Hopkins, who happened to be in the hospital, came in and checked on me. After listening to my chest and reviewing my most recent data, he suggested trying a cardioversion. A cardioversion is a procedure where two pads are placed strategically, one on the chest and the other on the back. A precise electrical shock is then delivered to the heart with the idea of converting an abnormal heartbeat back into a normal rhythm. My heartbeat at this point had become very weak and irregular and Dr. Hopkins thought it would be worth a try. The procedure was evidently successful enough for me to be sent home later that day without being admitted to the hospital.

In March, we had another clinic visit with Dr. Fowler at Stanford. He had previously made an appointment for me to have a Vo2 max test. It's a cardiopulmonary stress test designed to measure the amount of oxygen a heart can provide to the body's muscles during continuous activity. This test is considered to be a good indicator for informing cardiologists of the heart's capacity to keep a person functioning properly. The test involves the placement of electrodes on the chest and side, similar to having an EKG. The wires are then attached to a heart monitor and a blood pressure cuff is placed on an arm. My particular test was to be performed on a stationary bike. Sometimes the test is done on a treadmill. A soft rubber mouthpiece was inserted into my mouth. It felt as if I was preparing for a snorkeling adventure. The mouthpiece was attached to flexible tubing which was connected to monitoring equipment. A headgear apparatus was placed on my head for holding all the breathing equipment in place. A nose clamp was clipped on my nose and I was instructed to breathe through my mouth. A belt was secured around my waist for holding all the wiring in place. Now, I looked as though I was ready for a spacewalk. Next, I was instructed to begin peddling. The pace started out slowly with little resistance. However, the resistance and pace increased as the test progressed. All this time, I was only breathing through my mouth. With my condition as of late, I was worried I might not be able to go even a minute or two. I was asked periodically how I was feeling with the increased resistance? I was instructed to point to a chart and give the degree of difficulty I was experiencing. I also would give the okay or thumbs up sign. Much to my surprise, I continued for almost ten minutes. I worked up quite a sweat, my breathing towards the end became labored, and my legs muscles became very tired. However, I felt great afterwards, like I just had a good workout at the gym. There was no pain and I never noticed any weird sensations in my chest. When we arrived at our office visit with Dr. Fowler, he had already received my results from the test. He was very impressed with how well I had performed and was amazed, considering all my issues. We left the appointment on a high note and scheduled another appointment for a couple of months. Dr. Fowler stated that he would be in contact with Dr. Hopkins in regards to my good report. I had experienced some very low periods as well as some high periods. That seemed to be the way my condition behaved. That slippery slope thing almost behaved like a roller coaster ride. One day I was up and feeling well, and the next day, very down.

Experiencing more sleepless nights and constant coughing became a frequent routine. Sleeping medications didn't seem to help. My appetite was not very good and I was losing weight. After working all day, then attempting to eat dinner, the couch was my resting place until I could muster up enough energy to navigate the stairs up to bed. On one particular evening, we were in the family room watching television. The next thing I recalled was flying off the couch. It wasn't until a few seconds later before I realized what had happened. The defibrillator had shocked me! My heart had stopped! If it had not been for the defibrillator, I might have died. Lights out, the party was over. The shock felt as though I had been kicked in the chest by a horse. That was a common response, when asking other heart patients how it felt when their defibrillator activated. Questioning Dr. Hopkins' decision of implantation of the unit a couple of years earlier was very foolish on my part.

Sometime earlier, a defibrillator monitoring unit had been provided to me by Dr. Hopkins' office for the purpose of retrieving information which had been stored in the defibrillator. Accessing this information was done so by placing a mouse type device over my implanted defibrillator, just as had been performed on so many occasions in the doctor's office. This process could be done through any phone line, whether at home or traveling. After this episode, I immediately called Dr. Hopkins' office and was connected to the on-call doctor. He instructed me to transmit the data for review the following day.

Being placed on the heart transplant list had not happened as yet. We knew most likely it was to be very soon. Reading the literature which had been provided to us by Stanford had raised many questions in regards to how long we might have to wait after being placed on the list before receiving "the call" that a heart had been found. It could be as short as a few weeks, several months, or even up to a year. Once a patient receives "the call" there is a window of just a few hours for getting down to Stanford. The severity of a patient's condition and blood type often predicts the wait time. It is recommended a patient on the heart transplant list have a cell phone or a beeper with them at all times. It is never known when you might get "the call."

Another worrisome thought for me was the logistics of getting down to Stanford. We had a three to four hour window for getting there. By car, it was a two hour drive. I was worried my new heart would be waiting patiently for me in a cooler of ice and we would not arrive in time. Our friend's Jim and Donna's son-in-law Pat was an owner of REACH Helicopter Air Ambulance, headquartered at Sonoma County Airport, just north of Santa Rosa. Tentative arrangements were made with Pat that when we received "the call" from Stanford, all we had to do was drive to the airport. The airport was only a ten minute drive from our house. Upon our arrival, one of his helicopters would fly us to Stanford which was maybe a forty-five minute flight. Just the idea that that might be a possibility put my mind more at ease.

Easter was April sixteenth and we were invited to my niece Deanne's house for brunch. What I recall most on that particular Sunday was sleeping in one of her overstuffed chairs. I barely had enough energy for sitting up to enjoy her meal and participating in conversation with other members of the family. Looking back on those times today, I don't know how I continued trudging forward. I was miserable. Emotionally and physically I was not at all in a very good place.

Early morning Thursday, April 20, 2006, was to be the beginning of a whole new direction for my life. The evening before, Mary had once again taken me to the emergency room and again we were sent back home after a few hours saying there was nothing more they could do. After settling back into bed and falling asleep about one o'clock in the morning, I got up to use the bathroom at approximately 4:00 a.m. I walked into the bathroom, which was about ten feet from the end of our bed, and tried to sit on an upholstered bench which was in the middle of our bathroom/dressing room area. The next thing I remembered was lying on the floor between the bench and in front of our closets. Mary heard my moaning as I fell and came running into the room. I had passed out, fallen off the bench, and landed in a clump on the floor. I recall seeing feces all around me and I couldn't move any of my extremities. I was paralyzed and unable to speak. Mary thought I had had a stroke or a heart attack. She tried lifting me to get me back into bed with no success. I was dead weight and of course no help. I could hear her talking to me, but I was unable to respond. All I could manage was some mumbling. Mary called my sister Candi, who hurried over from across town. Mary had finished cleaning me up by the time Candi arrived. They assessed my situation and called 911. Mary and Candi were able to get me back into bed by the time the paramedics arrived a few minutes later. This whole event was a blur to me. I have somewhat of a recollection of being loaded on a gurney, carried down our stairs, and loaded into the back of an ambulance. I don't even recall too much about the stay in the emergency room. It was only after being moved to intensive care later in the day, before I was fully able to comprehend where I was and what had transpired. One thing I realized was that my defibrillator did not shock me. However, it was though my whole body was beginning to shut down. For several weeks prior to this most recent event, I noticed my self-catheterization process had been producing less urine. The weakened heart now was not providing efficient blood supply to vital organs. Sometime after being moved to intensive care, I was introduced to another new event in my life, kidney dialysis!

* * * *

Dialysis is the artificial process of removing waste and unwanted water from a patient's blood. When kidneys have been damaged or have failed, dialysis is the replacement of the function for which kidneys are not able to provide on their own. Without dialysis, toxins would build up in the blood and could eventually cause death. Kidneys help regulate the acidity of blood and control how much water is in the body. Stimulation in the production of red blood cells and regulating blood pressure are also important duties of kidneys. So when kidney function becomes compromised and you hear the term renal (kidney) failure, you might ask, what's next?

A catheter had been inserted into a vein on the lower right side of my neck, just above the collar bone. This allowed for access from the dialyzer into my body. Once I was hooked up to the dialyzer, the process for cleaning impurities would take three to four hours. During that time, the blood was being removed from my body, cleaned through the machine, and replaced back into my body. The size of a dialyzer is maybe the height of a three drawer file cabinet and has wheels for ease of mobility. The machine has a complexity of many gauges, dials, windows, and tubing. A technician would keep a watchful eye on the process as the dialyzer performed its function. After the three to four hour time period, I was unhooked from the machine and was good to go until the next time, maybe in a day or two.

Dr. Hopkins came into my intensive care hospital room saying it was time to get me down to Stanford. The time had finally come for the long anticipated heart transplant. I was scheduled for a transport ambulance ride on Monday morning. I just hung out in my hospital bed for the weekend with having another dialysis treatment, thinking about missing my niece Kelly's wedding, and reflecting back on a similar transport ride fifteen and a half years earlier. Even at this point, I still had not been placed on the transplant list. So my worries of not arriving at Stanford in time for the waiting heart was now no longer an issue. However, thanks to REACH Air Ambulance for being there if needed.

6
Memorial Hospital
2005—2006

Mary

Don's valve repair and defibrillator seemed to be working well. Then in the early winter months of 2005 things took a turn for the worse and we were referred to a Dr. Lee in Dr. Hopkins' office. Dr. Lee would be putting a third lead from the defibrillator to the heart. We were a little taken back by the office visit. Dr. Lee made it quite clear that this was only a "Band-Aid." He wanted us to know that this wasn't going to fix anything, just give us some extra time. The surgery was at Sutter Hospital where he had been many times before. So I waited patiently during the surgery in the waiting room for what seemed like a very long time. The doctor never came out to tell me how it went. But I will say that Dr.

Mundell, the anesthesiologist, who happened to be the husband of someone I had worked with at Steele Lane School, did come in and explained everything, telling me that Don did very well during surgery. I had been so worried and to this day can't thank Dr. Mundell enough for taking the time to set my mind at ease. I took Don home the next day and it seemed to me that he was doing better already. I remember telling friends at work that even though we had been told that the third lead was only a Band-Aid, it was the best Band-Aid Don had ever used. He was on cloud nine, doing all the things he had previously struggled with. He went to work every day, mowed the lawns, went for long walks with me around the neighborhood, which doesn't sound like much, but we live in a very hilly area of town. Even I sometimes got winded on our nightly jaunts.

Then sometime after the first of the year I started to notice little changes in Don. His skin was color was ghastly yellowish grey. He had trouble getting up our stairs to our second floor bedroom, sometimes having to stop two or three times to catch his breath. Our heating bill skyrocketed because we had the thermostat turned up to blasting. This was so much fun for me since at the same time I was having hot flashes, or what I referred to as "power surges" three or four times an hour. So as I was striping my clothes off, we were smothering Don in heavy wools and blankets.

During these first couple of months of 2006 we seemed to live part-time at Memorial Hospital's emergency room. I would bundle him up, get him into the car, and practically carry him from the car to the ER. They would tell us there was nothing they could do and send us home, where I would carry him back up the stairs. Many a night he would sit up in the chair trying to get some sleep to no avail. However, Don could fall asleep at the drop of a hat in the middle of a conversation with me or while watching television. One night while sitting on the couch with his back toward me watching the boob tube and me doing schoolwork at the kitchen counter, his head tilted to one side. I thought he was taking one of his many catnaps. All of a sudden his defibrillator went off. His body flew inches off the couch and he calmly said, "I think it went off." "It feels like a horse kicked me in the chest." I was nervous wreck, but Don went slowly to the phone to call the doctor's office which at that time of night was closed. However, the on-call doctor said he could either go to the ER or wait until morning to be seen in the office, which was what we chose to do.

Everything continued about the same until Easter Sunday. We were invited with the whole family to Don's niece's house. Almost the entire day Don slept off and on in her family room chair because he had no energy. He was so tired all the time and beginning to show signs of depression. All he ever wanted to do was to stay in bed.

About the same time, Don's other niece Kelly was getting married and Don did go with me to the dress shop to look for a dress. Unfortunately, he struggled to stay alert while I tried on a few. I got him home and he stayed in bed the next few days. This was the period of time where we were making our routine visits to the ER. So it was not a shocker when we had gone late one night about 10 p.m. and returned home about 12:45 after being told there was nothing more that could be done. Then about 4:00 a.m. I heard him call my name from the bathroom, but it was muffled. When I got to him, he was on the floor and couldn't talk. My first reaction was that he had had a stroke. He was dead weight and I couldn't lift him up even though he weighed only about one hundred forty five pounds at the time. Because I was in shock, rather than call 911 I called Don's sister Candi who drove right over. While I waited for

Candi, I tried to clean him up because he had soiled himself during the fall. When Candi arrived, she helped me get him into bed and we called 911. The paramedics, ambulance, and fire engine arrived in minutes. I think we scared the neighbors to death who thought Don had died. The paramedics were so calm and efficient. Two or three of the paramedics began working on Don right away and one came over to me to ask questions and tried to calm me down. I am sure when they saw all the meds on the night table next to Don's side of the bed, they must have wondered about overdose. I panicked when I overheard one of the men say he couldn't get a pulse and I started to hyperventilate. One of the paramedics asked me to take some deep breaths and put my head between my knees. They were all wonderful and whisked Don down the stairs on a stretcher and into an ambulance in a matter of minutes. The funny thing was that the ambulance left ahead of us for the hospital, but Candi and I arrived long before they did. They must have taken the scenic route and been in no hurry. It seemed as though it took forever to get him prepped and up to ICU. He had many visitors while being checked in including his niece Kelly, who was getting married that Saturday. Many of our friends also stopped by that weekend, which we greatly appreciated. Don remained in ICU until Monday morning before being taken by ambulance to Stanford.

Dr. Hopkins had come in to check on Don early Monday morning and informed us he had everything arranged for the transportation, all we had to do was wait for the call to move Don down to the ambulance. Everything was happening so quickly that I wasn't quite sure what my roll was anymore. So without thinking what it probably sounded like, I asked the doctor if I had time to go home and mow the lawn. He looked at me and said, "Priorities, Priorities." I then realized that it was a silly question, but did go home to grab an overnight bag for myself and rushed back just in time to follow the ambulance in my car down to Stanford. Don and I had been there many times, so we knew the layout and where the emergency entrance to the hospital was. However, this may have been the ambulance driver's first time taking someone two hours to Stanford. When they arrived at the hospital, they pulled into the front. I tried to motion to them that they needed to go around to the back. Eventually they figured it out and the hospital staff was ready and waiting for us in the ER.

7

Placement on the
Heart Transplant List

Don

Monday, April 24, I was loaded into the back of the transport ambulance for our two hour ride down to Stanford. Again, being all wired up with equipment, monitors, and accompanied by two drivers and a nurse, was very reminiscent of the Sequoia Hospital ride I had experienced some years earlier. However, this time I faced forward in the ambulance and was not able to see Mary following closely behind. Forgive me for borrowing a quote from Yogi Berra, the New York Yankees' hall of fame catcher. "It's like deja-vu all over again."

After arriving at Stanford late in the afternoon I was admitted through the emergency department and then taken directly to my room in the cardiology wing of the hospital. For the remainder of the week, and under the guidance of Dr. Fowler, I experienced a series of more screening, heart scans, blood work, and dialysis treatments in preparation for the transplant. Many of these procedures had been performed on me before. However, recent results would be needed for complete diagnosis and proper approach in accessing my individual transplant situation. By now, with all my crazy health issues, I felt I could be considered a professional at having medical tests and procedures performed, and can you believe, I was as yet to be placed on the transplant list.

Blood type is a key factor in deciding who is a good candidate for an organ transplant. Through all the previous years in dealing with my health issues, you would have thought I would have been aware of my blood type. However, it wasn't until the week of intense testing that I came to learn I was AB Positive, the universal blood type. It meant I could receive an organ donation from any other blood type. It opened the door for more possibilities of expediting the wait time for receiving a new heart.

During the week of testing, two recent heart transplant recipients stopped by my hospital room for a visit. Stanford encourages patients who have had heart transplants to share their experiences with people waiting for a new heart and to answer questions the prospective heart transplant recipient might have. The first was a man and his wife. He was a minister and she was a CPA. He was returning to Stanford that particular day for a follow-up appointment. They were a very gracious couple. Seeing how well they survived the experience and how the quality of his life had greatly improved, gave me hope that someday I might be telling someone of my experiences. The next person to share his story was a guy named Bob. He was a character! If I remember correctly, I believe he was a rancher from California's central valley. He said the doctors told him to get plenty of exercise. So he walked. He walked every day. He said, "You can't get enough walking in." The guy was almost fanatic about it. He also stated he performed arm exercises every day. He bought two one pound cans of corn and used those as his arm weights. Whether he was sitting in his lazy chair or lying in bed, he would arm curl those cans of corn. He also mentioned the importance of stickers. I remember thinking to myself, what is this guy going to come up with next? Stickers? When you get released from the hospital and return to Stanford for periodical clinic visits, patients need to pick up labels from the admitting desk before going to all their scheduled appointments. A label, or a sticker in Bob's case, was needed for lab work, echocardiograms, EKGs, chest x-rays, and clinic visits. The labels contained individual information for each patient. Of course, I didn't fully understand the label issue until months later, when I returned for my own clinic visits. Today, Stanford has changed from the sticker program to individual plastic identification cards which are presented at each clinic appointment. Trying to understand and comprehend Bob's dialog at the time was futile. Here, I hadn't even had the transplant as yet, and I had to listen to, "Don't forget your stickers." Even though Bob meant well, I was more than relieved when he finally left. I was never able to see the face of the minister or the man I now refer to as "Can of Corn Bob." They were wearing surgical masks, which were required for recent transplant patients.

Friday, April 28, after three days of intense testing, I was finally placed on the heart transplant list. Dr. Fowler came into my room and informed us that I had been placed on the list that morning. Now I felt there was light at the end of the tunnel. After years of office appointments, medical procedures, surgeries, and hospital stays, I was finally graduating on to becoming a heart transplant recipient instead of being a patient with congestive heart failure. I was being rewarded for all the years of perseverance. Sometime earlier, Dr.

Fowler had mentioned I would be the first patient with Ehlers-Danlos Syndrome to undergo a heart transplant at Stanford University Hospital. Even with Ehlers-Danlos being fairly rare, I was surprised upon hearing that information, since Stanford had been performing heart transplants for almost forty years. My waiting time could have been anywhere from a matter of days up to a couple of weeks. However, with having AB Positive blood type, my chances of a shorter waiting period was a strong possibility. Beyond the compatibility of blood types, there are other factors involved with qualifying a patient's eligibility for an organ transplant. A patient's life style, body weight, health condition and family support group, all play important roles in determining who is a good candidate for transplantation.

I eventually fell asleep late that Friday evening, after hours of contemplating what was lying ahead for me. My emotions were on overdrive with feelings of both apprehension and excitement. At approximately 3:00 a.m. the next morning, I awoke to a shadowy figure standing at the foot of my hospital bed. He said he was a member of my heart transplant surgery team and that a new heart had been found for me. I must have been dreaming or was it a nightmare, which was common place in a hospital setting. I said that I had just been placed on the transplant list the day before, only eighteen hours earlier. How can it be possible in locating a heart so quickly? The shadowy figure said sometimes hearts are found sooner than expected and that I had been placed very high on the list. He left with saying the team would be back in touch with me later that morning. I laid there for a while trying to absorb the impact of the information I had just received before calling Mary on her cell phone. I ended up calling Mary at about 3:30 a.m.

She was staying down the street at the SLAC House. She was almost in my room before I hung up. Mary called my son Mike, step daughter Tara, and my two sisters, Candi and Ardi, telling them the wonderful news. My sisters arrived by mid-morning and Dr. Fowler stopped by sometime later to inform us that Dr. Oyer and the team of transplant surgeons were assembling for their preparation before surgery and that they should be ready to go by early afternoon. Approximately two hours later I was transported to a heart transplant surgery room with my usual paraphernalia in tow; a heart monitor, IV bags, blood pressure cuff, and catheter. This was to be my big day, April 29, 2006. Mary and my sisters followed at my side all the way to the surgery room doors. Once again, one of the last things I remembered was Mary saying, "Think sex" and" I love you."

By the time I arrived in surgery, I was already groggy. Most likely I had been given something for relaxation. I was probably dreaming because I pictured myself as one of maybe a dozen heart transplant recipients all on operating tables waiting for our new hearts. Each of our new hearts were in sterilized individual stainless steel containers next to each of our operating stations. I could look over at my new heart and see it beating, all rosy red, just waiting for placement in its new home. The room was completely white with bright lights and every person in the room was dressed in white. However, I didn't notice any angels.

8

Two Transplants
in Five Days

Mary

Monday, April 24 through Thursday, April 27 was filled with testing, answering questions, and waiting for the doctors to come in to examine Don. We were both scared, anxious, and apprehensive all at the same time. Don was a nervous wreck the whole week so I would darken the room, ask him to close his eyes and think peaceful thoughts while I rubbed his feet, hands, and temples. I asked him to picture quiet beaches or sunny meadows while imagining the sounds of nature. We even had a masseuse come to the room one day attempting to relax him. While the masseuse was working on Don, I took a stroll down the hallway and happened to notice two ladies going in and out of a room just down from Don's. I later was told that one of them had a husband who had been waiting for three months to be put on the heart transplant list. Finally at 9:00 a.m. on Friday morning Dr. Fowler came in to give us the long awaited news that Don had been placed on the waiting list for a new heart. During the day Rodney Plante, our social worker visited with us to tell us all of the paper work, insurance forms, and Don's health care directive were in order. We were set to go!

About 3:45 Saturday morning Don called me on my cell phone to say they had a heart. I got dressed in about two minutes, left the SLAC House, and rushed to the hospital. I called his sisters to tell them the news, who arrived about 10:00 a.m. We all waited with Don until they came at 12:30 to take him to surgery. We were able to walk next to the gurney until we reached the surgery room doors, where I leaned over and whispered, "Think Sex." They informed us that the surgery would be about five hours, so Candi and Ardi left for home to avoid the commute traffic , while I remained in the second floor ICU waiting room. About 2:30 in the afternoon someone came in to tell me that they were going to wait for a different heart so the surgery was postponed for a couple of hours. It turned out that the original heart was better suited for another patient and a second heart was becoming available for Don, so we just had to wait. Then about 10:30 at night, Dr. Oyer came into the waiting room and told me the surgery went well and the doctors were just sewing him up. He said it would be a few hours before I would be able to see Don so I asked if I could go back to the hotel to get a few hours of sleep since I had been awake since 3:45 a.m. He said of course, so I left. One thing I neglected to mention is that everyone is asked to turn off cell phones while waiting in the heart ICU area. Thus, when I got back to my room, I fell asleep with my clothes on, and my phone turned off. I awoke to a sinking feeling that something was wrong. Realizing that my phone was turned off, I turned it on finding a message from the hospital to call a Dr. Oakes immediately. When I called, they told me to return to the hospital as soon as possible, nothing more. I walked to the ICU nurses' desk and as soon as I gave my name I could see a change in her face. She lead me to a small room and asked me to wait for Dr. Oakes. I should have guessed what the room was used for because there was one two-seater couch, a chair and three boxes of Kleenex. When he came into the room, I saw it written all over his face. All he said was, "It didn't go as well as we expected. There were some complications." I thought my heart had jumped into my throat. I actually had trouble breathing. He proceeded to tell me that the heart looked very healthy, but for some unknown reason it never started pumping on its own. They had placed Don on life support. He was alive, but not without mechanical help. They wouldn't let me see him right away, so I called his sisters who came right back to be with me. I also called Michael and Tara Anne, who rushed to the hospital.

There we made a vigil pacing back and forth in the hospital hallways. I joked that we were making permanent grooves in the flooring, but it wasn't far from the truth. The first night, Candi, her daughter Deanne, Tara Anne, and Michael stayed with me in my hotel room just across the street from the Stanford Mall and it was not too far from the hospital. We stayed up talking most of the night and I am sure wondering if we should be planning Don's funeral. I must say even though he was on life support, not once did I ever think he was not going to make it. We kept up the vigil until late on Tuesday night. We were sitting in the ICU waiting room about 7:30 p.m. when Michael got a call on his cell phone from Tara Anne who had just returned to her Pittsburg, California home earlier that day. She told Michael that Dr. M. had called to say they had found another heart. I screamed with excitement, but was puzzled because here we were outside the ICU doors and no one had said anything to us. Plus, I had my cell phone on and no one had called me. So I tore through the doors to the nurses' station and blurted out, "They found a heart for my husband?" She said she was very sorry but no one had called her so it was probably a mistake. Now we didn't know what to think. We waited and waited for what seemed like an eternity. Finally Dr. Oakes came out with papers for me to sign saying they had found a wonderful match for Don since he was AB Positive. They had a heart from a nineteen year old male from Reno who had been in an automobile accident. His wonderful family was donating his organs and we were the lucky recipients of his healthy heart. On Wednesday, May 3, after waiting all day with no more news, someone came out about 6:30 p.m. to say that the delay had been because Reno's operating rooms were busy all day and all the other teams of doctor's needed to meet at the same time for harvesting the organs. At approximately 8:30 p.m. they took Don from his ICU room into surgery with all his machines in tow that had been keeping him alive. One cute nurse told me she had never seen so many machines going into a surgery room. It added a little levity to the situation. However, Dr. M. was standing in the hallway with us as Don's bed was being taken out of room 13B and said, "You know he has only a ten percent chance of making it through this surgery. I was livid. I turned to him and said, "Why would you say that? Does it make you feel better? Does it help Don? Dr Oyer had just told us thirty minutes before that he gave Don a 50/50 chance , and we are going with those odds." He replied, "Well, Dr. Oyer is an optimist." I said I would rather go with an optimist than a pessimist any day. I still to this day have not forgiven Dr. M. What terrible bed side manners.

About 4:30 a.m. Thursday they brought Don out of surgery and Dr. Oyer informed us that Don had done just fine, but made me promise not to turn my cell phone off. We waited until 5:00 p.m. when they finally let us see Don, who looked terrible, but was alive with fewer machines.

The next days passed by slowly, very slowly, with very little change for Don. He had two nurses around the clock taking care of him. The nurses were outstanding! One told me that Don was taking "baby steps," but he was moving forward. On May 11, Rodney Plante called to say I was on the list for an apartment across the street from the hospital. There I could wait for Don's discharge from the hospital and subsequently joining me for his continued recovery and rehabilitation. It would be so much more convenient for me because of its proximity to the hospital, plus there was parking so I didn't have to search for a parking spot in the hospital garage each day.

9
Six Weeks in ICU

Don

My first recollection was Mary, Tara, and Mike smiling down saying how proud they were of me. What did I do? I was just lying there. How could I have done anything? I must have done something. But I didn't know what I had done. Why didn't they tell me what I had done? Were they trying to keep me from knowing something? Why was I the last one to know what I had done? In my stupor, I finally realized they were proud of me for not dying. I don't think I really understood what I had experienced and the fact that I had subjected my family to a long month of not knowing if I was going to survive. I had been placed in a medical induced coma from the end of April through most of the month of May. During that period of time I had received two heart transplants. I don't think Mary wanted to tell me what my body had been through. I finally learned through Dr. Fowler that the first heart transplant had not worked. The surgery had gone well, however the new heart did not begin pumping on its own. Dr. Fowler said the heart, which was currently beating in my chest, was the second transplanted heart. It was the end of May and after many days of questioning family, doctors, and nurses before I was able to sort out what had actually had happened to me. I remembered back to the unconscious patient who was in the bed next to me in ICU after my valve repair; the man who we thought was old with all the noisy equipment and waiting for a heart transplant. I remembered telling Mary at the time, I hoped that that was not going to be me someday. Well, in fact it turned out to be exactly my situation while waiting for the second heart transplant. From April twenty- ninth, following the first heart transplant surgery, until May fourth when I received the second transplant, I laid unconscious connected to the LVAD; left ventricle assist device. Doctors were unsure if I would be able to stay alive long enough to make it to the second heart transplant. I learned months later the family had been discussing plans for my funeral. I fooled everyone.

My recovery was very long and arduous. After coming out of my unconscious state, I remember laying there in a bed, not knowing where I was. A nurse or a doctor asked me if I knew my name and if I knew where I was. I tried to say my name was Don, but I didn't know where I was. I thought I was in Santa Rosa. They informed me I was at Stanford University Hospital in the intensive care unit. I remember not being able to speak and was hardly able to move my arms and legs. With the ventilator down my throat for so long, it took me some period of time after its removal before I was able to effectively communicate and be understood by those around me. I realized early on after regaining consciousness that I wasn't able to talk. Not knowing I couldn't swallow, I tried desperately asking for a sip of water using the limited amount of sign language I was capable of. Also, I wanted to know if Dr. Oyer had been in to see me. However, I couldn't get the words out of my mouth. My attempt at speaking sounded like mumbled garble. Finally, one of the nurses got a chart with letters of the alphabet on it. I pointed to the "O" and then the "R". Everyone thought I wanted orange juice. I shook my head no and kept pointing to the same two letters. After several frustrating attempts and with tears running down my face, they eventually realized what I wanted. In my stupor I was pointing to the "R" instead of what I should have been pointing to, which was the "Y". I am certain if I had pointed to the first two letters of his name in proper succession, everyone would have known I was asking for Dr. Oyer.

My kidneys had pretty much shut down and I had been on 24/7 dialysis during my unconscious state. What little urine I produced had the consistency of molasses and the color of dark coffee. The thought was that possibly the kidneys might improve within a couple of months. Nephrologists would keep a watchful eye for improvement. Often, as we learned with congestive heart failure patients, when a heart fails it can also take the function of the kidneys with it. This appeared to be my predicament, but we held out hope that with time there might be a return to better kidney function. If I had received a new heart a few months sooner, then possibly my kidneys may not have been as dramatically affected. It all goes back to the slippery slope that Dr. Fowler talked about early on. There was that fine line between being okay and falling off the ledge.

With time, my ability to speak slowly returned, but I was still unable to swallow liquids. Now, doesn't that sound silly? Everyone swallows! That's a natural reflex, right? Well, in my circumstance I guess it wasn't. With kidney failure and dialysis, I was constantly thirsty. I would have done almost anything to get my hands on a nice cold lemonade. But, then what would I have done? Each time I attempted swallowing even a little water I choked and coughed and spit it back out. Until the swallow reflex returned, the nurses were hesitant in allowing me any more attempts at swallowing, instead they would give me flavored pink swabs on white plastic sticks for creating moisture in my desert dry mouth. I guess for the time being I had to be satisfied with the expectations that someday I would once again be able to have that frosty lemonade.

Since I was not in a position for taking any nutrition orally, a feeding tube had been inserted through my nose down my throat and into my stomach. An awful substance called Nepro hung in a bag above my head with a constant flow of the stuff into my body. I needed nutrition for helping with the healing process and Nepro seemed to be the best choice and met the nutritional needs of patients on dialysis suffering from kidney disease. The stuff was tan in color and appeared to have a consistency similar to that of a milkshake. We learned that Nepro was a hospital version of Ensure. The problem with the Nepro treatment was it would flow out of my body almost as quickly as it went in. It was almost like _ _ _ t through a goose. I was constantly being cleaned up. Often, no sooner than being cleaned up I had to ring the nurse again. This vicious cycle went on for weeks. I am sure the nursing staff got very tired of the routine, however they always seemed pleasant about it.

Slipping to the bottom of the bed was another constant occurrence. With the head of my bed somewhat elevated, my body would slip toward the end of the bed. With not having any strength in my arms and legs, I didn't have the ability to push myself up, so I was always requesting the nursing staff to pull me back toward the top of the bed. My doughy and stretchy Ehlers Danlos skin didn't offer enough resistance against the hospital bedding to keep me in one position. If they had tied me to the wall, that might have alleviated my problem.

Through the heart transplant ordeal my body weight dropped down to a skeleton like 103 pounds. I was like a rag doll and barely able to lift my arms. Mary and the nurses would exercise my legs. It was almost as though I was paralyzed; a vegetable just lying there. I needed help in sitting up and had to be held so not to fall over. Nurses would pick me up and place me in a chair next to the bed and tie a flannel sheet diagonally across my chest. I was petrified at this process, thinking I would fall over and land in a clump on the floor. I was so weak that while being tied to the chair I could hardly lift up my head. My head would flop down with my chin resting on my chest.

Thinking back to my friend "can of corn" Bob, I asked for a couple of small cans of Nepro from food services. The cans were probably only eight ounces of liquid, however they offered just enough resistance for doing curls with my withered arms as I laid in bed. A peddle contraption on a stand was brought into my bed area for exercising my legs. Much to my surprise, as well as the doctors, I was able to proficiently peddle, although still being tethered to the chair. With performing the arm and leg exercises, I slowly began regaining some movement in my limbs. However, sitting upright on my own was another issue. It took months of therapy before we saw much progress in that area. I had no core strength after lying prone and enduring the two heart transplants and frequent kidney dialysis. I was so weak I couldn't have fought my way out of a wet paper bag. I may have had a new healthy heart, but the rest of me was still a work in process.

My bed in ICU was an area of constant activity. A speech therapist was assigned to me with a program to help strengthen my vocal cords. Daily respiratory and breathing treatments were administered by respiratory therapists to help my lungs rebound from the pneumonia and collapsed lung that occurred during my month long sleep. A hand held pounding unit was used daily against my chest and back by therapists. The pounding of this machine was to help with breaking up the infection. Every morning began with chest x-rays, where a technician would bring a portable x-ray unit to the side of the bed for taking my daily picture. Nurses would be taking vitals, checking monitors and IVs, administering my daily anti-rejection drugs, and making sure the Nepro was flowing properly. It seemed as though I was constantly receiving medications around the clock for one thing or another. Throughout the day there would be a constant stream of doctors coming in for short chats. Often professors would bring their medical students, interns, and senior fellows by for case study and then quietly disappear. Early on in my recovery, I would be transported at least once a week in my hospital bed to the cath lab for a heart biopsy, which would tell if I had any rejection with the new heart. A tiny piece of tissue would be snipped from the heart and sent to the lab for study. Visits were also made to the echo lab, which of course I had become very familiar with during my years of care with Dr. Hopkins.

Hallucinations were a common occurrence during the nighttime hours when I should have been asleep. Sleeping soundly I guess was just not a part of my program. One would think after what my body had experienced for the past several weeks, I would be sleeping continuously. I probably slept more during the daytime than at night. Those nighttime hours dragged on for ever with crazy night-mares torturing my mind. Some examples of such was; a movie be-ing filmed in ICU with the doctors and nurses in staring rolls. The premier of the movie was going to be held upstairs and of course I wouldn't be in attendance because I was busy as an emcee of a tele-vision game show. My nighttime nurse sat at a table at the end of my bed doing school work since her day job was a school administrator. A model train ran around the perimeter of the ICU on the ceiling. I could hear the conductor say, "All Aboard," and the whistle blow as it passed over my bed. My brother-in-law, Ed Meyer, stopped by at the end of my bed and conducted a fight song with his spirit team from his college days at Notre Dame. In fact I asked Mary if she had seen her brother before he left. Now, doesn't that all sound rather silly? However, it certainly seemed so real to me at the time.

I was one of four patients in our intensive care unit. There was a bed next to me and two beds across the way which were divided by a glass partition, and I was visually aware enough to see what was happening in my confused world. My roommates would come and go. They would be there for a few days, then they'd be gone and new patients would come in taking their place. This scenario played out for several weeks with me becoming more upset and agitated as the days dragged on. I was still there and they all returned home, or so I thought. With seeing how upset I was, Mary whispered to me, "You know Don, you are probably the healthiest person here." At the time I don't think I grasped the meaning of her statement. It was some time later before I understood what Mary was trying to tell me. Some patients did get moved on to other rooms and eventually returned home, however many of my bed mates had died. I guess I was one of the healthiest patients there and very lucky to be alive. I could have been on my way to the morgue. My outlook towards the continued stay in ICU had suddenly changed. I was one of the very lucky ones!

After becoming aware enough to understand I had been unconscious for most of the month of May, I realized I had forgotten that Mother's Day had come and gone. I felt badly that I wasn't in any condition to get Mary a Mother's Day card, so I asked one of the nurses if she would go downstairs to the gift shop and buy a card. The only problem was, I didn't have any money. She said that was okay, "It's on me." Since it was already past Mother's Day, the only cards she could find were for Father's Day. I must have spent at least an hour trying to write "Dear Mary and Love, Don" in the worst and almost unintelligible hen scratch you could have imagined. Even though it was difficult for Mary to read, it brought tears to her eyes knowing how hard I worked on it.

Sunday June 18th was Father's Day and it was quite a special day for me. Our children, their spouses, and grandchildren all came for a visit. My atrophied, withered, and fetal positioned body was strapped into a wheelchair for a ride outside to the fountain area in front of Stanford Hospital for a family picture. Being part of a world I had not experienced during the last couple of months was a refreshing change. With a cowboy hat on my head that Mary had bought for protection against the warm, sunny day and the surgical mask around my face, no one could enjoy my exuberant smile. After my ride to the great outdoors, we all came back to a waiting room in the hospital, which happened to be closed that day, to open my Father's Day presents. My dexterity still was not the greatest, so I needed help with trying to remove the wrapping paper from the boxes. One of the gifts was a white t-shirt from Tara, Spencer, Janae & Garen which said in black letters, on the front of the shirt,

"I Left My Heart at Stanford," and on the back, also in black it said, "But They Gave Me A New One." What a great gift! I knew at that moment if someday I was ever to write an accounting of my health experiences, I already had a title.

After being aware and comprehending all the physical trauma that my body had been exposed to, I became inquisitive as to what had happened to my original heart. One of the reasons for my curiosity was wanting to see what my enlarged heart looked like in comparison to a heart of normal size. We were informed that hearts which had been removed for transplants were kept in the lab and would remain there for a period of time. I asked Mary Burge if we could take a wheelchair ride to visit my original heart. She responded positively and said she would look into making the arrangements. We inquired several times but because of paper work, vacation schedules, and my therapy regimen we could never coordinate the proper timing for the visit. I had to be satisfied with the mental image of my old heart floating in a large pickle jar full of formaldehyde.

10
Getting Into a Routine

Mary

On Friday night, May 12, the most wonderful thing happened. I walked into the ICU room and Don had his eyes open, not for long, maybe ten seconds, but it was a start. They had stopped his sedation medication two days before and now he was beginning to wake up. That night I said goodbye to Don, the nurses, and the rest of the people in the room. The next morning when I arrived the three other beds in Don's room were empty. I asked the nurse where the other three patients were. She just shook her head and said they did not make it. I went over to Don's bed and leaned down to whisper in his ear, "Honey, you are the healthiest one here."

The next day Candi and Ardi came to visit. When they walked into the room, they were met with an astonishing sight, Don's head was propped up and his eyes were open. He still had the breathing tube in, but he tried to talk. He asked for water, which was still a no, no. He really didn't talk. He put his thumb and pointer finger together to make a sign for "a little bit." I had previously taught him a few sign language signs. We could somewhat understand his attempt at signing, however it took us quite a while to figure out that he wanted a little bit of water. Shortly after his sisters left, Tara Anne brought our granddaughter Janae to see Don. It was so exciting because the nurses allowed us to bring Janae up to the window and lift her up so she could see Don and he could see her. The hospital did not allow children in the ICU so this was the closest we could get her to Don. He smiled and showed he was able to recognize us. Up to this point we were never sure if he knew who we were. On this visit, Tara took a picture of Don with her cell phone so hopefully someday he could see how much he resembled the Michelin Tire Man. The nurses had Don's arms and legs continually wrapped with quilt-like blankets to absorb the fluids that were secreting from his extremities because his kidneys had stopped functioning. They exchanged these blankets every couple of hours when they became saturated. I have no idea how much he weighed at this time since he was mostly water weight.

Tara Anne and Janae stayed with me at the Country Inn Motel that night. It was sort of like a slumber party. Tara shared the bed with me and we had a trundle bed brought in for Janae. It was my fifth motel since coming down to Palo Alto, but it had a kitchen and a pool, so it was well worth the drive. I was still waiting to hear for an opening at the apartments across from the hospital. It would be about the same price as the motels, but closer and bigger. The reason Tara and Janae had come to visit was because Sunday, May 14 was Mother's Day. We all went up to see Don for the ten o'clock visiting time. For the past month I had been referring to the visits as "viewings" because Don would just lay there with no response and me doing all the talking. Even when he had his eyes open, it was like he was looking right through me, not really registering who I was. It was difficult saying goodbye to Tara Anne and Janae when they left to have Mother's Day in Pittsburg. She had brought me a beautiful framed picture of the whole family taken at Christmas, pictures of Janae and Garen, and a huge Mother's Day balloon. She had also bought the makings of dinner on Saturday night and made me a great chicken parmesan dinner which I found out later was paid for by Rob and Jen as my Mother's Day gift from them.

On Sunday afternoon Mike came to see Don and watched the Giants loose to the Dodgers. It was probably a good thing that Don couldn't keep his eyes open because he is usually swearing at the TV during a Giants telecast. He was on his sixth consecutive day of dialysis and they had started feeding him through his nose, thus he was zapped of all energy let alone trying to stay awake. We left him about dinner time since it was a pretty good guess he didn't realize we were there anyway.

On Monday, I got to him at about eight-thirty a.m., he had his eyes open for about ten seconds and that was it. He didn't seem to recognize me. They had him on a very slow drip of nutrition through his nose and a respiratory specialist was giving him a dosage of anti-fungus medicine through his mouth, however Don couldn't close his lips around the tube to breathe it in so the nurse had to use his hands to close around Don's mouth. About this same time guess who came in? Dr. Doom and Gloom. Dr. M. walked up to the bed, took about fifteen seconds to look at Don, and said he was surprised Don was doing as well as he was. He turned around and walked out. Don told me later that he liked that doctor, but I am so happy I didn't have to deal with him again. Dr. Oyer came in about 5:45 that evening to say they were going to start feeding Don intravenously besides through the nose to the stomach. I hoped this would give him the energy he needed since he would be starting speech and physical therapy soon.

We had another set-back! The next morning when I got to Don, the nurse informed me Don's right lung had collapsed during the night. They were going to give him a breathing treatment (a mask) that would help his lung to expand. They had to do it at night because the mask was extremely uncomfortable. About noon, our friends Jim and Ted called to say they were at PF Changs, so I met them for a wonderful lunch. Ted treated and their visit got my mind off Don for a while. We all went back to see Don, who had his eyes open and seemed to recognize us. He even attempted a half-hearted wave and tried to say in a garbled voice, "Hi Ted." I left that night to drive back to Santa Rosa for a doctor's appointment with my family doctor. I don't know if it was from all the stress I was going through or if I had caught a bug in the hospital, but I had the worst case of diarrhea and nothing I took seemed to help. I arrived back at Don's room Wednesday afternoon. He seemed alert but couldn't talk and was very raspy in his breathing. The nurse tried to get mucus out using a suction apparatus, but didn't get much. He was very weak and had to use his stomach to breathe. Each breath was a struggle. About 3:30 they asked me to step out of the room. At 4:00, Christine Hartley called me on my cell phone while I waited in the ICU waiting room to tell me Don needed a breathing tube put back in because he couldn't breathe on his own. They had given him a sedative to allow him to rest, so I left for the night.

By this time, I had gotten into a rather mundane routine. Each morning I would rush to shower and race to the hospital to see Don before the night nurse had left so I could ask her how he had done the previous evening. This was usually before 7:00 a.m. because they switched shifts each morning at 7:00 and the nurses needed time before visiting hours to relay the night's information to each other. After I saw Don, I would leave the ICU North and walk down the back stairs to the cafeteria that was on the first floor by the entrance to the emergency room. Just as you get down the stairs, there is a Starbucks. It became my home away from home. Every morning I practically ran to the Starbuck's line to get my chai tea and sometimes a blueberry muffin. Then I would walk back upstairs to wait in the ICU waiting room for the first visiting time of the day. Don't ask me why, but on Thursday, May 18, I took a different route to get back upstairs. I walked to the front of the cafeteria to head up the main stairs of the hospital to the second floor. Little did I know that I was about to encounter something that would change my life and my routine for most of the rest of our stay at Stanford. I was about half way to the stairs when I heard the most beautiful music coming from the atrium in the hospital's basement floor. It was someone playing show tunes on the piano and I followed it like a moth to light. I continued following the sound until I saw who it was. He was all by himself and seemed to be oblivious to anything or anyone. I sat down in a chair next to the windows behind him, listening, and finding myself transported to a magical place. Forgetting about how lonely, depressed, and scared, I had been. I just sat and let him take me to a calmer place. It turned out that I would from that day on check to see if he was there before going upstairs each and every day. Sometimes I would just sit and listen and sometimes I would bring my knitting. He wasn't always there, but when he was, he would nod to me and continue playing. It wasn't until weeks later that I even worked up the courage to ask him his name. He told me his name was Lawrence Mathers and he was a physician in the children's hospital next door. He had a habit of taking his breaks there with the piano. I told him I appreciated how much his music helped me to relax, but I don't know if he really understood what a lifesaver to my emotional being his music was all those months. Between his beautiful music and the Bing Music Program at lunch time on Wednesdays and Fridays, I felt I had some sanity to my life.

On that same day, when I got to the hospital, the nurse said Don had sat up on the side of the bed the night before for a few minutes with the help from the physical therapist. However, it was difficult for me to believe because he was so comatose all the time. I was never completely sure if Don knew if I was there or not. That same day our friend Rosie called telling me Kristine, her daughter and Jason were expecting. That night I told Don the great news and he flicked his eyes open which told me he understood what I was telling him. The hospital was trying to get more nutrients into him to get him stronger so eventually he could breathe on his own. He still looked yellow because his liver wasn't working well. The swelling in his hands, arms, legs, and feet was getting better, but was still bad considering he had been on dialysis for nine days. We had been at Stanford at this point for weeks, and it was still difficult for me seeing Don in this condition. He was a trouper and had been through so much. It made me love him more and more every day. The kids and our friends were so good about calling me every day to see how Don was doing. I appreciated their love and caring.

On Thursday and Friday the doctors decided to try Don on every other day dialysis. This meant Don would have a technician come in, hook him up to the dialysis machine, and dialyze him for three to four hours a session. We all hoped that he would be able to adapt to three days a week rather than the 24/7 machine that he had been on. Tara, Spencer, and the children came to see him on Saturday. The nurse informed us Don hadn't done well on the every other day sessions of dialysis, so they would be changing him back to the 24/7. This was discouraging for us because we considered this a setback and it meant having that huge noisy machine back next to his bed, once again inhibiting our ability to get up close. One thing Don thoroughly enjoyed was anyone gently rubbing his arms and legs. So during this visit, that is exactly what Tara did, and to our amazement, Don opened his eyes a few times.

They had hooked him up to 24/7 dialysis by the time I got back from 8:45 mass on Sunday at St. Thomas Aquinas Church. Don didn't open his eyes much for me throughout the day, but he did when Mike and Julianne arrived at about 6:15. The three of us went to dinner, talking about Don the whole time. When we got back, the night nurse, whose shift began at 7:00 p.m. and who was new to working with Don gave us more information than we had ever received. She said he could go either way. James, who was Julianne's brother's respiratory therapist, was in the hallway when we were leaving and told us to be patient.

When I got there Monday morning, Deanna, who was Don's nurse the day before, told me that they had stopped giving Don the Dopamine and his oxygen was at 16% support. He seemed more alert and smiled when I called his name. He had his eyes open for longer periods throughout the day. In the afternoon, Dr. Oyer and another doctor came in to see Don. I was in the waiting room, so I missed seeing them. However, the other doctor came back and told me they were going to slowly decrease Don's oxygen until he could breathe on his own, keeping the ventilator in just in case he had trouble. However, if he couldn't breathe without the ventilator, they would have to perform a tracheotomy. I almost started to cry, but the doctor assured me they would try everything else first. When I left to go back to the motel, Don lifted his right hand and tried to wave to me. I never told him about the possibility of a tracheotomy because he had enough on his plate already.

On Tuesday morning I arrived to find out they had changed him back to the three hour dialysis. Deanna said he was doing well, but they needed to watch his breathing, which he was doing on his own with 12% support. If he could continue this way, the tracheotomy would not be necessary. Dr. Oyer did come in to say there still was a chance he would need one, but they would give him some time to see how well he could do on his own. His liver was better, his skin color was no longer orange/yellow, and he did a little better on dialysis. Things were looking up!

Don had at least 16 different roommates in the bed next to him by the window. One of these patients was a little short Jewish lady with a great sense of humor. She was extremely gregarious and even showed me her tattooed number from the concentration camp on her left wrist. When I was going to leave that night, she said, "You're not going to leave me alone with your husband, are you? You don't know the trouble the two of us might get into." When she was moved to another room, I asked if Don could be moved to the window bed and Deanna said, "Why not?" This was after I had asked three or four other nurses who all said, "We don't move patients to other beds." I understood how difficult it was to change all the information from one bed to another for the same patient, however, Don had been looking at walls and dividing curtains for weeks and I felt that the ability to look outside and see some light would do wonders for him emotionally.

Sally was his nurse on Wednesday, May 24. I liked her a lot.

She exercised his legs and was extremely gentle with Don. They took him off the pain medications and sedatives, so we just had to wait until he woke up completely. If he became more alert, they would remove the ventilator the next day. They started a feeding tube through his nose hoping it would give him energy to make it easier for breathing on his own. Candi, Ardi, and Deanne came about 5:30 p.m. and took me out to dinner after seeing Don. They were all teary-eyed, but thought he looked better.

On Thursday, May 25, I had to leave Don shortly after lunch to drive to Santa Rosa for some errands. We had had the mail stopped and collected at the post office where I periodically had to pick it up. I also planned on going to my elementary school's open house that night to meet with the parents. Before I left Don's room, a social worker came in to tell us Blue Cross Insurance had okayed all the bills, not that they would pay it all, but at least the charges were all accepted. It was up to the hospital and the insurance company to negotiate the bills. We had been told it was over one million for a transplant. We could only imagine how much two transplants and months in ICU would be.

When I arrived back the next morning shortly before 11:00 a.m., the nurses were nice enough to let me in an hour earlier than the usual visiting time. My friend Lorol arrived shortly after that and I brought her up to ICU to see Don. Lorol was there to see her friend Laurie, who was having an x-ray down in the cancer wing. The three of us went to lunch and shopping. Lorol had brought me a tote bag with five novels, a bottle of wine, and her homemade coffee cake. She is always so thoughtful. It was uplifting having her drive all the way down to see me.

The next day when I arrived at 9:00 a.m., Don looked better and there wasn't as much swelling or yellowing of the skin. They had just started dialysis and the technician said everything was going well. They ended up taking 3.8 liters of fluid off Don, which was the most in any one day. At 10:00 a.m. I returned to his ICU room and noticed his head was very clammy, but Sharon, his nurse said it was nothing to be concerned about. However, by 4:00 p.m. she told me his whole body had been sweating for the past two hours and his numbers went plummeting. They gave him some kind of shot and he was fine shortly thereafter. The doctor had just checked him and said Don was stable after being given a mild sedative. Sharon said it scared everyone because Don was considered the healthiest of the four roommates. Through all this turmoil Don flicked his eyes open only a few times that day.

I went to 7:30 a.m. mass on Sunday, then went to Safeway to get some junk food for a picnic that I was going to have later with my children, then fixed breakfast at the motel before getting to Don at 9:00 a.m. He looked so much better, had his eyes open, and was able to visually follow me around the room. Jolan, who was his nurse that day, said he was doing well with his breathing. His lung was still collapsed, but much better. They would skip dialysis for that day because his numbers looked great. Dr. Laversen came in with three other doctors and said Don was slowly getting better, but needed to be fed more. It turned out that about 4:00 in the morning Don had started thrashing with his hands and had pulled the feeding tube out of his nose. They were waiting for x-rays to see if the newly placed tube was in the correct spot in his stomach. When I got back at noon he was being fed once again with Nepro. I liked Dr. Michael Laversen who was from Holland. He was always so positive and would talk directly to Don. Michael, Tara, Spencer, and the children got to the hospital about noon that day. We stayed and chatted with Don until 12:30 p.m. when we left for the picnic and a swim back at my motel. While we were gone, Don watched the Giants baseball game when Barry made home run #715. When we got back to the hospital, Don said he saw the home run, but everything else we asked him, he couldn't answer. He started getting agitated. Jolan made a chart with the alphabet written on it, but Don wasn't able to point to the specific letter of the word he wanted to convey. He started getting frustrated, so then Mike and I started getting frustrated. When we told Don we were leaving for the night, he started to cry and shook his head "no."

The next day was Memorial Day and once again Jolan was Don's nurse. He was so gentle exercising Don's legs and arms plus cleaning him up when the feeding tube leaked. When I got there at 8:00 that morning, Don was alert and a little agitated. He cried every time I left the room. The hospital allowed us to visit in the ICU for fifteen minutes at a time every other hour starting at 10:00 in the morning. Because I had been there for so long and was pretty well acquainted with most of the nurses, I was allowed a lot of flexibility with this routine. If I wasn't in the room with Don, I was usually found in the ICU waiting room with the other family members of ICU patients. One day a Catholic priest came into the waiting room to give communion to those who wished to receive. Two women beside myself received and so we started a conversation. It turned out that Pat's husband was the one waiting three months to be placed on the heart transplant list. Kathy was her sister, and later the three of us became good friends. I stayed at the hospital until 8:30 when Jolan said he was pretty sure they would be taking Don's ventilator out sometime late that night or early the next morning. He had had dialysis late that day so they had to take him off the feeding tube while on dialysis. Don was becoming stronger each day and we all hoped that he would be able to breathe on his own soon. Even though his improvements were slow in coming, Don was doing better than a lot of other patients. The man who was across from Don in the next room was going to lose his toes through amputation. He had no circulation so his toes had turned black and hard. The only way to stop the progression of the gangrene was through amputation. We felt so lucky and so proud of Don for hanging in there and keeping a positive attitude.

The next morning I had a little shock. When I walked into Don's room, the bed was empty. The nurse saw the expression on my face and told me that Don had been moved to room nine which was just down the hall. I walked in and almost didn't recognize him without the ventilator which had been removed the evening before, after I had left the hospital. He was sitting up (propped) and talking. It was the best present that I could have ever received. Joy, his nurse, said he was doing well and I could see for myself how great he looked. Our friends Jim and Donna called that morning to meet me at Café Barrone on El Camino. It was their anniversary, so I suggested to Don that we practice saying the words, "Happy Anniversary," to surprise Jim and Donna when they walked into the room. But when I asked Don to practice he started to get tears in his eyes. This was the first time that Don realized this was the end of May and the whole month of May had slipped by. Don had remembered it being April when they took him in for the first heart transplant and didn't realize until now that a whole month had passed.

Ellen Mundell, who was the wife of the anesthesiologist that assisted with Don's third lead procedure back in Santa Rosa, and worked with me at school, came down to see Don and take me out to lunch. We went to the California Café, which was not too far from the hospital. We sat and talked over a couple of glasses of wine. This little outing was exactly what I needed instead of having lunches alone in the hospital cafeteria. Mike and Julianne came later that afternoon and stayed until about 6:00. While Mike was in the room, the physical therapist came in and asked him if he would help her hold Don up in a sitting position with his legs over the side of the bed. He sat there (with help) for a good five minutes. The speech therapist, who happened to be partially deaf, also came in to do exercises with Don. Don was doing well, improving daily, and becoming more mentally alert. He was getting his speech back and it was much easier to understand him. He wanted, "Out!"

I went to Santa Rosa on Wednesday and returned Thursday, June 1, late in the morning. Don was fast asleep. Cathy, who was his nurse, said they were going to do dialysis and a biopsy that day. Each procedure individually had the capability of zapping all energy from Don, so it was difficult to understand why they would consider performing both on the same day. They did do his breathing treatments and dialysis that afternoon, but no physical therapy and no biopsy. Laurie came in at 3:00 and said they had to wait until the next day for the biopsy, speech therapy, and physical therapy. That was just fine because Don had no energy to stay awake anyway. It seemed to be a struggle just to keep his eyes open. Don's sister Candi called and asked if she could come with Ardi to see him on Friday and I said yes because it might perk him up and help me because I was feeling bad. When I arrived at the hospital that morning, they told me Susan's husband had died the night before and the older gentleman who had taken Don's bed in 11B had also passed away. I was so happy that Don was doing better, but it was difficult to meet so many people, become friends, and share their grief. Later that afternoon I walked over to my friend Pat's apartment at the Oak Creek Apartments. It was so beautiful overlooking a creek with meandering paths down below. The apartment had a huge master bedroom and a sunny living room. I was so jealous, but I knew I could never afford the $3,650 per month and a six month lease. She had the option of staying at the H.O.M.E. Apartments, across the street from the hospital, but chose Oak Creek.

Dr. Laverson, Dr. M, two other doctors, and Christine Hartley were all in Don's room when I arrived on Friday, June 2. They were all saying how well Don was doing and Christine said they were shooting for Monday to transfer Don to room D3. Rodney Plante came in and said there still was no room for me at the apartments across the street. I asked how soon I could take Don home. He looked at me like I was crazy and said, "Do you realize how serious your husband's condition still is? He is going to be here for months." If Don was going to be in the hospital for months, it was real important for me to get into the apartments as soon as possible. Rodney left, then returned about fifteen minutes later, saying there was an apartment available for me. I was so excited I could have done jumping jacks. Instead, I left immediately to check out of The Country Inn Motel and check into the new apartment. I had to wait until 2:00 to check in. When I got there, the manager was late and showed another woman a big apartment on the first floor, got her all checked in, and then showed me mine at 3F. It was terrible. It had an air conditioner right up to the side of one of the twin beds and it was a lot smaller than the one I had seen downstairs. The more I thought about it, I wasn't happy, so I asked if I could be put on a waiting list for a better room. She said she had another room, 2G. It wasn't anything spectacular, but I took it. This would be my home away from home for the next four months.

Once I moved into the H.O.M.E. Apartments, my routine progressed at a smoother pace. I was able to go back and forth to the hospital at my will rather than spend my hour and forty-five minutes in the ICU waiting room or in the atrium downstairs. The H.O.M.E. Apartments is an acronym for Housing of Medical Emergencies and is operated by the Assistance League of Santa Clara County. The H.O.M.E. is for out-of-town patients and their families while receiving treatment nearby at Stanford Hospital & Clinics. The apartments were funded by the Flora Lamson Hewlett Foundation and were originally opened in 1987.

On Wednesdays and Fridays, in the atrium from 12:30 to 1:30 they had wonderful music programs that were put on by the Bing family who also donated all the artwork down the hallways and all the beautiful flowers and their maintenance in the gardens surrounding the hospital entrances. Now that I was settled in so close to Don, I could run back to the apartments for a quick swim and be back for his next visit. Most days were filled with reading hundreds of books, knitting, or taking long walks around the campus in between the bi-hourly visits with Don. And some days were filled to the max such as Saturday, June 3. I started out driving to Walmart, which was quite a ways to drive, to get some needed things for the apartment. Then I visited with Don until our friends John and Janet arrived about 10:30. They were pleasantly surprised to see how well Don was doing. The three of us went shopping in the Stanford Mall and they treated for lunch at P.F. Changs, which seemed to be a favorite place for many of our friends. While having lunch, we got a long distance call from Lorol who was in Hawaii. I was a little jealous and would have easily left in a heartbeat to join her. Getting back to Don about 4:00 p.m., I found him in great spirits, but asking for a foot massage and to exercise his arm and legs. Early on in ICU Don had leg wraps on both legs which expanded and contracted with air for the stimulation and circulation of his lower extremities. Don was constantly asking for the wraps to be removed because they caused his skin to perspire. Thus, after having them removed, he still enjoyed his legs and feet massaged.

After grabbing a quick dinner and a change of clothes, I walked back to the hospital at 8:00 p.m. I couldn't say 8:00 "viewing" anymore because he was talking more and more, actually trying to have a conversation. That night I finished wrapping birthday presents for Garen and putting together the dinosaur costumes I made for the children's party he was having the following week.

I was so proud of how well Don was doing physically and how positive his attitude had become. At the same time, it was equally difficult for me to see my friend Patricia going through such a trying time. The doctors had told her there was no hope for her husband. He had been waiting for a heart transplant for months and because of his health history, his size, and blood type, they had run out of time. She had been told that it was necessary for her to sign papers for his removal from life support. I don't know if I could do that. It takes a very strong person. Even when Dr. M. told us there was only a ten percent chance of survival, I never thought that Don wouldn't make it.

Don was waiting for me and perked right up when I arrived about 9:00 after mass on Sunday, June 4. I had gone with Pat and Kathy who were coming to grips with the decision to stop all life support on Pat's husband. Don seemed better, but the nurse said he had been coughing all night. Two doctors came in to say he had to pass the swallow test before he could be moved to the intermediate ward. Then to add insult to injury, the nephrologists came in to say his kidneys were still not working, though they had not lost hope that his kidneys would start producing urine on their own in a couple of months. Dialysis had been ordered for Sunday and Monday.

Michael and Julianne got to the hospital just after lunch and visited with Don for about an hour. They then drove me to Tara Anne's house for Garen's birthday party, which was wall to wall dinosaurs. They got me back to Don at 7:30 so I could visit for a couple of hours. It turned out that Pat and Kathy were visiting at the same time and invited me to join them for mass the next morning at 7:15, which was being offered up for her husband. It worked out perfectly because Don was so tired from all the Sunday visitors, that it allowed him to sleep in on Monday.

When I got to Don on the morning of June 5, he was extremely depressed. The doctors had just left and Don had not passed the swallow test. I tried to cheer him up by telling him that it was one of those tests that you are able to take over and over until you pass. Little did we know at that time that he would be taking it over and over. Unfortunately, because he didn't pass it this time, he would not be allowed to move to the intermediate ward and they wouldn't be administering the swallow test until the following week. Shortly after that, Dr. Laverson came in to say they needed to take Don to O. R. to have a permanent catheter in his neck for his dialysis.

By noon, my two good friends Rosie and Marylou arrived. I met them downstairs and as we walked up to see Don on the second floor, I tried to prepare them. I said he was very weak, thin, and had trouble talking. But when they walked in, I saw how shocked they were. They stayed for the visiting time, but Rosie got all teary eyed when she left the room. I knew then that I had made the right decision when I told the rest of our friends to wait to come down to see Don until he was better. The three of us went to lunch and shopping at the mall. We were window shopping when I got a phone call from a doctor who said he was in Don's room and I needed to get back to the hospital immediately to sign papers giving permission to do the procedure for the catheter. I said goodbye to my friends, rushed back to the hospital, and then waited until 10:30 that night. They never came to get Don. Finally, one of the nurses ran to the cath lab to see if they were still on for the procedure only to find the place shut down. I guess it's the old adage; hurry up and wait. While I had been having lunch with the girls, a therapist had Don sitting in a chair for almost thirty minutes, the longest so far. However, with that physical therapy, dialysis, and the anxiety of waiting for the catheter surgery, Don was exhausted, so I left him sleeping soundly.

Up until now everything had been going along pretty smoothly in regards to my interactions with doctors, nurses, therapists, other patients, and their families. It becomes a fairly close-knit community when you are there practically 24/7 for weeks and weeks. When I got to the hospital on Tuesday, June 6, that all changed. Walking up to the nurses' station about 8:00 a.m., I asked Natalie to call into Don's room to see if I could pop in for a quick visit, something I had been doing every morning for at least a month. The nurse on duty said, "Yes." However, when I walked in, the nurse told me my shoes were too loud and dangerous. They were the very same shoes I had been wearing every day for the last seven weeks and no one else seemed to mind. They were little slip-ons with one-half inch heels made out of rubber. At 11:00 a.m. they took Don to O.R. for the placement of the permanent catheter in his neck for his dialysis. He came out at 12:15 and had done beautifully. Tara Anne, who arrived at 10:00 that morning stayed until 2:00. After saying good-bye to her, I returned to the room to see Don, where the same nurse proceeded to criticize everything I did. She told me I had to leave when Don was just about to have physical therapy, which I had been waiting to witness for the last three to four days. Don started to become agitated asking for the same male physical therapist that he had the day before. Don was still leery of his own lack of strength and with his fear of falling, he felt more at ease with this gentleman. Upon hearing this, the nurse told us she was more than capable of holding Don up on the edge of the bed, "I'm the nurse, you're the patient." The more agitated Don became, the more she started yelling at Don. I am embarrassed to say it, but I blew up, really lost my cool, and told her she needed to work on her bedside manners. I shouted that she may be a great nurse, but her social skills stunk. It turned out that the news of my outburst reached Christine Hartley, who was the head nurse. She could not have been sweeter. She told me that they would be putting a different nurse with Don and that sometimes there are personality clashes that need to be worked out. Most of the staff bent over backwards to make Don feel less stressed and I am sure that I was under a lot of stress myself, so the slightest provocation was going to send me over the edge.

That evening they told us that Don would probably have to remain in ICU for another two to three weeks. You can imagine how well that went over with Don and me. His potassium level was 6.5 and should have been below 5.0, so more frequent dialysis was needed. I left the hospital exhausted about 6:30 p.m. to heat up leftover Chinese food and to listen to the harpist who was playing on the third floor of the apartments. Once a week the Bing Foundation paid for entertainment for the patients who were recovering at the H.O.M.E. Apartments.

Wednesday, June 7, was quite a day! I didn't go in to see Don until 10:00 a.m. Kim, who was Don's new nurse was very nice and very pregnant. They were doing dialysis and a breathing treatment at the same time. So the PT (physical therapy) girl said she would come back, which she did about 12:00. She did some great exercises with Don and with help from Yvonne, the deaf speech therapist, got Don sitting up on the edge of the bed for ten minutes. He complained how tired he was, but I was so proud of how well he was doing.

When I arrived back at 4:00, Kim said he didn't pass the swallow test for the third time, but she showed us some exercises he could do with his mouth, tongue, and neck to help with hopefully passing the swallow test next time. Also at 4:00, Pat and Cathy pulled the plug on Pat's husband. My heart dropped. I know it was selfish, but they were my salvation every day. I didn't have anyone else that I was close to at the hospital. Eva was taking her husband home on Friday and Joe and his mother Melinda left the previous week. Don was depressed when I first got to his room in the morning, but seemed to cheer up after the PT left. She told us, for every six days you are in bed, it takes six weeks of therapy because you lose one-half of your muscle every six days. Don really worked hard with the exercises because he wanted out of ICU worse than I did.

Because it was the end of the school year, I wanted to go back to Santa Rosa to say good-bye to the class I had left in April during spring break. I left on Thursday, June 8 to spend two days cleaning out my classroom, saying good-bye to everyone, and making an appearance at the end-of-the-year party at Barry Kelly's, our principal. It was so great for my morale to see the children, who bombarded me with hugs and kisses. After working all afternoon in my classroom, I went to our house to pack up some things to take back to the H.O.M.E. apartment, such as some extra dishes, kitchen gadgets, and extra linens. Michael was visiting Don that day and called me that night to say Don had sat up for forty minutes. On Friday, I finished the clean-up in my classroom and left Santa Rosa before lunch time.

I stopped at Don's work in Petaluma to pick up an enormous poster that Audrey and Lisa had made with all the Kresky employees' pictures. It was a huge hit in ICU. Don was having dialysis when I got back and the nurse had just weighed him at 104.9 pounds, which was up over a pound from the last weigh-in. His nurse was Liz Marie and she told me Don needed to go in for another biopsy at 4:00 to see if there was any rejection with the heart. When he returned to the room two hours later, they had given him pain medication and he was extremely tired. His new catheter for dialysis was not in all the way, so they scheduled Don for another ride to the O.R. on Monday. Because they happen so often, we didn't think twice about these procedures anymore.

On Saturday, Don's nurse Laura, with help from Carlos the PT, got him sitting up in the chair from 11:00 to 12:15. He started to complain at about 12:00, but she asked him to hold out for fifteen more minutes and Don said, "Okay." His speech was getting so much clearer. The nurses were optimistic about getting him moved out of ICU by Father's Day. Unfortunately, Don was getting a little discouraged that he was still so weak, so he pushed himself even harder when it came to the exercises that were given to him. He did tell me he thought he was breathing better, another big improvement.

Another discouraging development was when they moved his roommate Kevin to an intermediate room that night. Don got so upset seeing patients coming and going in a constant parade while he remained glued to his portion of the room. Now that he was able to comprehend what was going on, he had to fight the frustration. We talked a lot about taking him to P.F. Changs for lemonade, taking him for a stroll outside in a wheelchair, and getting a full body massage; all things that would have to wait.

After mass on Sunday, June, 11, I arrived to see Dr. Laverson talking with Don. He told us that it was extremely important for Don to pass the swallow test before being allowed to move from ICU to intermediate. The doctor said he had to be honest, it didn't look like it would be before Father's Day. Then in an instant, that proves the right hand doesn't know what the left hand is doing, the night nurse, Pat, said she heard they were shooting for the next day to move Don. It surely perked up Don's spirits. When I got back to him after lunch, he was sitting up in the chair bicycling away with no effort like he was preparing for a marathon. The PT said she would bring a half-pound can for Don to use for arm strengthening. She also gave him some new exercises to help his shoulder muscles.

Nothing much happened on Monday. Don continued with his exercises and I had a few visitors. But Tuesday, June 13 was a great day for news. Linda, the case worker, came in the afternoon to say Don's bills had reached the seventh highest at that time in Stanford's history, and Blue Cross was going to pay everything so far except three-thousand dollars. We worried that our lifetime cap of five million dollars with Blue Cross might be in jeopardy. Don and I agreed we would deal with the financial issues when the time arose. Don was supposed to have a new pic line put into his left arm that day, but they never came. He was also scheduled for another swallow test, but they never came. He did sit all by himself at the edge of the bed and dangled his feet. I was impressed with the big improvement in his capability. Don started talking about the possibility of taking early retirement. I thought it was a great idea, but in the same vein, he talked about how much he missed work and the people at Kresky Signs.

* * * *

Wednesday brought another swallow test and another failure. Because he aspirated, they wouldn't let him leave ICU. Our children were planning on visiting for Father's Day so I asked Valerie, his nurse for the day, if we would be allowed to put Don in a wheelchair and wheel him out of ICU to see the kids if we strapped him up well, put a paper mask on for protection, and didn't keep him long. She thought it would do him a world of good. Then, the breathing therapist said his lungs were sounding a little better, but his right lung still hadn't expanded enough, so they were continuing with his breathing treatments. These sometimes consisted of having him breathe medicine through his mouth, then using a vibrating machine on his back to loosen the congestion in his lung. Also that day, they started catheterizing him in hope that his kidneys would start producing some urine.

Our friend Denny sent a lovely card to Don, his first received at the hospital. It cheered Don so much that I called her to say how much he appreciated it and I would let her know when he could have visitors. I didn't want a lot of people seeing him yet. I thought he looked great, but experiencing how some reacted to his state of condition, told me he needed a little more time to recover. Little things started to bother Don. He was discouraged how slowly his energy was returning, that he couldn't pass the darn swallow test, and that night, his nurse was a huge man from Barbados who Don said scared him to death.

We had another tremendous day on Thursday, June 15. Christine Hartley came at noon to take Don for a wheelchair ride. She first put him in the chair, then secured him in with flannel sheets pulled diagonally across his chest and tied in the back. We placed a big hat on to protect his head from the sun and of course the paper mask over his nose and mouth. She rode him around the big water feature in front of the hospital. He watched the ducks until he complained of becoming tired, but upon returning to his room, he exercised on the foot bike. The nephrologist, Dr. Scandling came in that evening to tell Don the kidneys didn't look good and we were probably looking at dialysis for rest of his life. I thought Don was doing so well, but it was discouraging for me to see how frustrated Don still was. He was getting crankier to some of the nurses who really tried their best and were oh so gentle with his care. We just had to get him out of ICU before we both went stir crazy.

The next day Don was still depressed with his lack of progress. I kept telling him that he should have seen himself six weeks before, all skin and bone. Christine came in and said Don would be moved in three days, on Monday, to D3 where he would remain for three weeks. He then would be hopefully transferred downstairs to the rehabilitation wing, where he would have therapy every day for three to four hours. At that time, they would be teaching both of us about the administration of his numerous drugs.

Our friends DiAnn and Terry came down to see Don and take me to lunch. When we got back at about 2:30, Don was sound asleep, so I said good-bye to our friends and took a swim. It was June 16, and it was ninety-five degrees in the shade. However, when I got back to Don at 4:00, he was furious with me that I hadn't been there with him all day. When I left for dinner, he panicked that I wouldn't come back. He had another attack when I had to leave at 10:15 that night. We were definitely looking forward to the intermediate ward where there wouldn't be such strict visiting hours. Plus, having a private room would allow me more flexibility.

The day before Father's Day was Saturday, June 17 and my

son Rob, his wife, and their three month old daughter arrived from southern California in the afternoon. We all walked over from the apartment to see Don, which boosted his spirits. His nurse, Justin got him into a wheelchair so we could take a short walk around the hospital. All of this seemed to put Don in a much better mood than the previous few days.

Father's Day was great! The children were there and we all went outside to have Justin take a family picture of us. After that, we had our little family party in the waiting room around the corner from ICU. We all helped Don unwrap his gifts; a picture of Mike and Julianne from Mike, two hearts; one chocolate and one toy from Rob, and from Tara Anne, a shirt that said, "I Left My Heart At Stanford" on the front, and on the back, "But They Gave Me A New One."

11
Intermediate Room

Don

Finally, by that third week of June, evidently I had improved enough to be moved to an intermediate room on the third floor of the hospital. Maybe the Father's Day celebration, being with family, and a bit of fresh air provided a jump-start to my next level of recovery. The swallowing problems continued. My kidneys had not improved. The dark color and syrupy consistency of my urine remained the same as it was in ICU. Nephrology didn't think the kidneys would ever come around, however with more time and dialysis, we would see how it played out. The good news was that my new heart had shown no signs of rejection. The periodic biopsies in the cath lab had always indicated zero rejection. Of course, we were ecstatic hearing that information. Knowing the heart was healthy and performing as it was supposed to was always great news.

Now, if we could only get the rest of my body parts and other organs to fall in line, we would be home free. Rejection can be a problem with any transplanted organ. A transplanted organ is considered an outsider in its new home. Not being a part of the original equipment, the body's defense system wants to throw it out, trying to eliminate this new foreign object. One might say the body is prejudice against these new intruders. The answer to this problem is the introduction of anti-rejection drugs. Transplant patients will take anti-rejection drugs daily for the remainder of their lives with the hope of providing insurance against rejection.

The intermediate room was a private room, which was a nice change after all the daily commotion down in ICU. I had my own suite and now I could entertain in style. The room had two chairs, a closet, a nice sink, and a roomy bathroom. It was almost like being at the Ritz compared to ICU. If only I was able to get out of that darn bed. Well, I guess I wouldn't have made for a very good host anyway, due to fact that my swallow reflex hadn't returned and the feeding tube remained through the nose and down my throat for administering the awful Nepro. While in the intermediate room, doctors decided to have the Foley catheter removed from my bladder, which had been in place for the past two months. Leaving a catheter in place for a protracted period of time can increase the chances of infection. Being immune suppressed, which is a side-effect from taking anti-rejection drugs, the chances of getting infections become many times greater than a patient who has not had a transplant. So with removal of the catheter, my immune compromised body had a better hedge against infection. Dialysis treatments in the intermediate room had been reduced to every other day. Since I still wasn't producing very much urine anyway, nurses could straight cath me on the days I didn't have dialysis. However, nurses had difficulty with insertion of the catheter into my bladder while I was lying in the prone position. I felt it was probably something to do with my weird connective tissue disorder; Ehlers-Danlos Syndrome. I asked the nurses if there was some way they could sit me up in bed and swing my legs over the side. With them supporting me, I would be upright and in a better position for performing the catheter procedure with my own hands. Nurses wheeled a contraption into my room which was a lift that had a leather strap for placement under my rear-end and straps for positioning across my chest. I sat in this harness thing which they then would crank up, placing me in a standing position with most of my weight being supported by the lift. I was sure this kind of thing was used for paralyzed patients. I might as well have been paralyzed because I wasn't able to sit up or stand on my own. Once in the standing position, I could then perform the catheter process as I had done thousands of times before. So those days on which I didn't have dialysis, became my peeing days. What a lot of trouble to go to the bathroom!

12
Physical Therapy

Mary

My son, Robert and his family had to leave on Monday, after Father's Day, but it was a full day for Don anyway. Don slept most of the morning after having a biopsy. Then he had dialysis from 2:00 to 5:00. At 5:30 they moved him out of ICU to intermediate D3, room 323. PT never seemed to connect with him because of his busy schedule. I loved his new room. It was private, had a view of the front walkway and gardens, plus it was extremely quiet. Another great thing about his private intermediate room was the pullout chair that converted to a flat bed. I spent many hours listening to my iPod while Don took naps. I even spent a night or two, although I woke up as stiff as a board.

On Tuesday, June 20, his first full day out of ICU, he was doing so well. I had called a few of our friends and told them the direct telephone number to Don's room and some had already called. One of these calls was from Jim, who had been such a savior for us. He not only went over to our house twice a week to check and mow the lawns, fixed the broken sprinklers, but he made sure to run the car periodically so the battery didn't die on us, something I never thought of. We owed him big time. A few of Don's doctor's came in that day to say they had two huge concerns. One was the lack of kidney function, but the first and main concern was the inability to pass the swallow test. Don was still getting breathing treatments and his blood pressure was going up. The good news was that they felt he was strong enough to begin going downstairs by wheelchair for dialysis rather than by transport gurney, which he had been doing since entering the hospital.

Wednesday was a busy day. I got to Don at 7:30 a.m. and shortly after that, PT came to work with him. Then two from speech came to say they would try another swallow test on Thursday. Next, transport came to take him for chest x-rays. From there, they took him down to dialysis from 12:00 to 4:00. No sooner had he returned to the room, respiratory therapy came to give another treatment. By this time, Don was a wreck and asked for a Xanax. We watched Jeopardy on his TV while I did some arm, leg, and throat exercises with him. Don was thoroughly exhausted, but perked up when Michael called shortly before I left for the night. Little things like phone calls and short visits perked him up beyond words.

Thursday, June 22, brought yet another failed swallow test. But the physical therapists, Cory and Shelley brought a contraption into Don's room to help Don stand up. It was the weirdest thing I had ever seen. They put strapping under Don's bottom and across his chest. Then with Don sitting on the edge of the bed, they cranked him up to a standing position, something he had not experienced for two months. Later that afternoon, Debbie, the speech therapist, came in to say they felt strongly about putting a feeding tube into his stomach because Don had not passed the swallow test. Both Don and I felt we were between a rock and a hard place. On one hand, we wanted that stupid feeding tube out of his nose, but on the other hand, we were petrified of the exposure to the infections a stomach tube would introduce. The doctors who came in that day all agreed we would be discussing it more thoroughly. Then that evening, the night nurse tried to catheterize Don with no success. This meant that he would be taken somewhere where they could find out the problem. On a lighter note, we were notified Don qualified for rehabilitation and as soon as an opening arose and he passed the swallow test, they would ship him downstairs to the rehab wing. Rehab was exactly what he needed to get back on the road to recovery.

Friday was the same old thing, with x-ray, dialysis, and PT. I stayed all day with him. Then when he was watching the Giants on TV and half asleep, I tried to leave and he got all upset. The separation anxiety was becoming a constant issue.

Audrey and Steve from Don's work came to see him on Saturday, June 24, right after he finished an hour of PT. It was tremendous for Don to see someone from his work. They got him smiling when talking about the old and new employees. Plus, I think they were pleased to see Don had their poster displayed on the wall of his room. As they left, Mike and his girlfriend came. The three of us worked to get him into the wheelchair for a ride around the grounds. One of the places we took him was to the outside seating area for the cafeteria. It was cruel, but we sat eating sandwiches and drinking liquids while Don sat looking on. I could almost see him salivating.

Sunday was a rough day, I even placed sad faces next to my journal entry. It started off well with me taking Don for a ride around the hospital, back to ICU for a visit, and the Linx restaurant. However when I got him back, the nurses wanted him standing up in the contraption from the other day to get a urine sample from him. Everything came out looking like black coffee and was such a small amount. That didn't work, so they put him back in bed on his side. Not only didn't that work, but his feeding tube got accidently pulled out and had to be reinserted twice. Then he was x-rayed twice to make sure it was correctly placed. The reason they needed an un-contaminated sample of urine was because they were pretty sure he had a bladder infection. When you are on anti-rejection meds, your immune system becomes compromised, thus the introduction of infections. The good news through all this hassle was that Don had the feeding tube out for a short while and told us that he could swallow. We hoped that they would leave it out for good, but it wasn't in the stars. Don was so tired from the feeding tube and the swallow tests that I thought he would cry.

About a month before, I had met a gentleman in the ICU waiting room whose wife was having lung problems. Charles and I became friends and after his wife was discharged, they came to see Don periodically. On this particular day when Don was feeling really low because of all he had been through to get the urine sample, they came to see him. They meant well, but they told Don about their friend who had a stomach feeding tube for over two years. Right after they left, Don started to cry uncontrollably. He couldn't imagine being strapped to eating this way for ever.

Don's dialysis lasted from 8:00 a.m. to 1:00 a.m. on Monday, June 26. No sooner did he get back to the room and I had to leave for a meeting. Stanford has a wonderful service in which they gave support to the care givers of transplant recipients. They met one day each month and answered questions or gave advice to those who either had someone waiting for a transplant or just received one. It was all so helpful to me who felt like a fish out of water. Everything was new and scary for me. The meeting that day, from 1:30 to 3:30, was led by Mary Burge, the transplant coordinator where I met a man who had once played for the Grateful Dead and was waiting for a heart. He was so upbeat, telling us that he probably would never get a new heart for a number of reasons; his blood type, he was overweight, his age, and he had used drugs. But he remained positive that he would live his life to the fullest. We met another gentleman a few months later at these meetings, who was an airline mechanic. He and his wife moved from Hawaii to be closer to Stanford in case a heart became available. He had been waiting for quite a while due to the fact that his blood type was O and could only receive from a donor with O blood type. Don and I saw them the following Christmas at one of our follow up visits and he told us he had received his new heart the week before. What a Christmas gift!

After that day's meeting I rushed back to Don's room, but was told he had been taken at 3:00 to the cath lab for a biopsy and to have a new pic line put in. They said he would be back at 4:00. He arrived back at 6:30 and was exhausted. He did get a visit from Father Hester, the Catholic priest for the hospital. He had a calming effect on Don and promised to check on him again even though Don wasn't Catholic.

On Tuesday, June 27, someone came in with a smaller wheelchair they had borrowed from the children's wing of the hospital. Not only was it a better fit for Don's tiny body, but they had placed a four inch foam pad in it to make for a more comfortable ride since he had no meat on his rear end. Don had two great phone calls that day. One was from his childhood friend Tom, who got him laughing and promised to stop by soon for a visit. The other call was from our next door neighbor, Don, who said he had some wonderful relaxation tapes for Don to listen to while lying in bed. The next time I went back home, I picked them up and they were perfect for soothing Don when he became agitated.

Our friends Ted and Lorol came on Wednesday, took me to lunch in downtown Palo Alto, brought homemade oatmeal cookies, and gave me a dress and Don a shirt from Hawaii.

But the best gift was the meditation tape that Don began using right away. They must have known how badly his spirits had sunk, because it was exactly what he needed.

On Thursday, I stopped in to see Don early in the morning because I was going back up to Santa Rosa to get mail, run some errands, see friends from school, and have an appointment with the head of human resources for Santa Rosa City Schools. I needed to talk to him about where I stood with my job. My accumulated sick days were running out and if I took leave of absence, I wanted to make sure I would have a job to come back to. He couldn't have been nicer about it. He assured me that I had enough to worry about with Don and I would definitely have my old place back in first grade. I showed Ron pictures of Don taken on Father's Day. I could tell he was shocked in seeing how thin and gaunt Don had become, but I assured him I would be back teaching in a few months. Little did I know at that time it would be five months later.

When Don got back from three hours of dialysis on Friday, they tried to get him on to a standing scale to weigh him and he had a fit. I don't know if it was partly because he didn't want to actually see how much he had lost or if he just didn't have the energy to stand up alone and was afraid of falling. They finally gave up trying. When the speech therapist came in to have him try swallowing tiny ice cubes, he surprised us. Sometimes he could swallow with no trouble, then again the next time, it would go down the wrong way and he would cough and it would come up with gobs of mucus which he couldn't or wouldn't swallow. Thus he depended on the suction tube he had been given. Don would panic if he didn't have this tube in his hand or a least close by on the bed. My dream was just to get him off that suction apparatus and relax enough to swallow on his own. They were still talking about moving him to rehab the next week, but not if he hadn't passed the swallow test and/or break free on his dependence of the suction tube.

On July 1, he was supposed to have a visit from his friends Vern and Don, but they called to say they couldn't make it. Norm and Patti also called to say something had come up and they would not be able to come. Then Tara Anne called to say she had to meet a prospective buyer for their Jeep and would try to see Don the next weekend. To be honest, Don handled it pretty well saying how tired he became when he had too many visitors. So I took him for a ride to the Rodin sculpture gardens and around the Loop and past the church on the Stanford campus. What a beautiful church! There was a wedding going on that day so we didn't go in. It turned out to be a very sunny day and I was afraid of keeping him out in the sun too long. They told us over and over how susceptible Don was to skin cancer due to the anti-rejection drugs he was on.

On Sunday, July 2, Mike met me at the hospital after I had picked up some lunch at Drager's (my favorite place at the time). When we arrived at Don's room, he was already in the wheelchair so we rode him over to the apartments, just one block over. It probably sounds cruel, but Mike and I ate our lunch in front of Don again. He was okay with it and was happy to see the apartment for the first time. We got him back to his room just in time to watch the Giants game. Watching baseball gave him a little respite from the depressing realization his recovery was going to be slow, a lot slower than he wanted.

All the previous week Don was taken in the morning for dialysis. Wouldn't you know it, on Monday, July 3, when friends were coming down, his schedule got switched to the afternoon. Norm and Patti did come that afternoon in time to see Don for five minutes before he was whisked off. After Norm and Patti took me to lunch and left, I waited until 5:45 for Don to return from dialysis. I left in the late evening to try to watch the fireworks display. The next morning he told me he enjoyed hearing them from his bed. The following three days were basically the same routine.

13
Rehabilitation

Don

One afternoon, while I was still in the intermediate room, a doctor stopped by introducing himself. He stated that he was the coordinator of the rehabilitation wing of the hospital and that my team of doctors thought I would be a good candidate for admission to the rehab program. He said they would be studying my complicated case and a decision would be made by the following week to see if I qualified. After staying in the intermediate room for only two and a half weeks, I graduated on to the rehabilitation wing on July 7. I felt lucky to have been accepted and maybe my ability for recovery would finally get kicked into high gear. After languishing for so long in ICU and with only a short stay in the intermediate room, now things seemed to be moving fast. However, the transition process was very frustrating for me. I was asked a battery of questions pertaining to my records. I felt I had to explain my health history every time I changed rooms or whenever there was a shift change with the nursing staff. Upon settling into my new room, I was asked where my list of medicines were. I said they were in the red binder which had been provided during my stay in intermediate. I also said they should be in their computer system. That's not something a patient should have to be responsible for and in my already agitated state of mind, I became even more upset at the situation. I think part of the problem was the hospital was in the process of going on line with a new computer system. During my stay in intermediate and then in rehab, nurses and staff were so over-whelmed with the training of this new program, it appeared to me they were overburdened while trying to contend with their regular duties. Eventually my binder was located.

My room, being another private room was the first room in the rehabilitation wing, right off the main hall on the ground floor of the hospital. The room was bright and airy with a nice window looking onto a walkway lined with beautiful summer flowers. The walkway was one of the main entrances to the hospital and adjacent to the cafeteria which had an outside dining area, so I could watch people coming and going throughout the day.

In my particular hall of the rehabilitation wing, there were prob-ably five or six more rooms just like mine, with patients needing re-hab from the results of accidents, amputations, and surgeries. At the end of the unit was a large therapy room filled with an assortment of equipment; several adjustable platform beds, arm and leg peddle machines, parallel bars for assistance in learning to walk, a tread-mill, a stationary bicycle, and a stair/step platform. If I had to attach a term to my time spent in rehabilitation it would be, "Boot Camp."

My days once again began as they had in ICU and in the inter-mediate room with a buzz of early morning activity. After things had settled down, Ryan, one of the physical therapists, would come to my room, for the morning therapy session. Early each morning one of the nurses would post a list of my daily activities on the wall in my room, placing me on notice as to what my program was to be for that day. My first thought was, "I am going to have to do all that?" Ryan just had his hands full trying to get me sitting up in bed, then swinging my legs over the side and adjusting the height of the bed so he could slide me over and into the wheelchair. After that, I was exhausted and we hadn't even made it to therapy yet. In the beginning, I wasn't much help with this undertaking, however after a couple of weeks, I was able to offer some assistance for our daily trips down the hall. I had both morning and afternoon therapy sessions.

After arriving in the therapy room, I was taken to one of the adjustable platform beds. Ryan would once again lower one arm on the wheelchair, adjust the height of the platform bed, then slide me on to the platform while supporting my back into a prone position. Whew! Once on the bed, one project was knee bending exercises. While Ryan created resistance with hands and arms, I pushed against the resistance with each leg individually for sets of ten. That wasn't too bad. Another project was trying to get me to stand. Ryan would wheel me on to the parallel bar platform, then grabbing hold of the bars with each hand, one bar on the left, the other on the right, I was supposed to pull myself up to a standing position, (I was lucky even to be able to hold on to the darn bars). My arms, legs, and back were just so weak that I couldn't do it. Other attempts at standing had me sitting on the edge of the platform bed with the height adjusted so that my legs were touching the floor, almost in a standing position with the weight of my body mostly supported by the bed. A walker was then placed in front of me while Ryan stood in front holding the walker. I was then instructed to grab hold of the walker, again trying to pull myself into a standing position. I was still unable to perform as instructed. My legs were so wobbly they wouldn't support me. Also, I was petrified that I would fall over, crashing to the floor, even though Ryan was right there to catch me if that should happen. These attempts went on for weeks before we saw much improvement. I guess rag dolls don't have much strength in their limbs. By the time I arrived back in my room from the twice a day workouts, I was completely spent, as though I had just run a marathon. My weight at this time was still only a whopping 110 pounds and having basically no core strength, any attempt at these simple physical tasks were next to impossible.

My daily training would alternate between physical therapy and occupational therapy. Those sessions would always have to be worked around my every other day dialysis schedule and my periodic visits to the cath and echo labs. If I had physical therapy in the morning, then in the afternoon I would have occupational therapy. Occupational therapy sessions began with learning how to get dressed and putting on shoes. I will tell you, at this point physically, I was still not a whole lot passed being a vegetable. It was suggested that I wear exercise clothes and tennis shoes for my daily workouts. So Mary picked up a couple of skinny outfits for me at the Stanford Mall. Occupational therapists showed me techniques on how to get dressed while lying in bed and the use of assist devices for putting on socks and shoes while sitting in the wheelchair. Once in the therapy room, therapists would have me perform a series of arm strengthening exercises, one of which was the use of the peddle machine which I peddled with using my hands and arms. Therapists would also have me perform hand exercises such as; squeezing a small rubber ball, lifting my arms over my head one arm at a time, and board games for improving my finger and hand dexterity. I excelled quite well with the assigned hand and arm exercises, however, when it came to standing, or with any movement that required strength in my legs and back, I was done. I still couldn't sit up without the support of a chair at my back.

The most frustrating aspects of my rehabilitation were; not being able to swallow and the inability to stand. Ryan worked many hours trying to teach me the technique for getting into a standing position from both the platform bed and the wheelchair. I always felt I was going to topple over and land on my head when attempting to stand. We as healthy, strong people often overlook the mechanics involved with our ability to stand. We just do it without thinking. It's automatic. Due to the fact I was always in fear of falling forward, I would attempt to push myself straight up from the sitting position with just the use of my arms. Of course, that's not the way we do it. It's almost impossible to push oneself into a standing position with just your arms, even more so if you don't have any strength in your legs for assistance. Try it sometime, it's very difficult. The way I finally learned the mechanics of this difficult process was to have me lean forward while holding on to the walker and pushing up with my thighs. At the same time I was to straighten my knees and back, thus forcing myself into a standing position. We lean forward when we stand and leaning forward was my obstacle. With my fear of falling and without proper strength in my legs, we worked for weeks before I gained enough strength and confidence in re-learning the mechanics of how to stand. Once I conquered the ability to stand, the next frontier was learning to walk. Oh boy! With my weak legs, I was faced with yet another challenge. We first started with me going to a standing position from the wheelchair while Ryan held a walker in front of me. Next, I would grasp the walker attempting to take steps down the hall toward my room. Ryan would follow closely behind, pushing the wheelchair as protection in case I was to fall or needed to take a rest. Early on with my walk training, the approximately one hundred feet from therapy to my room seemed to be a mile. In my weakened condition and with becoming extremely out of breath trying to perform this difficult task, I would have to stop several times falling back into the wheelchair to rest before proceeding. We practiced this routine daily, eventually gaining the strength and confidence needed for successfully negotiating the way back to my bed. Another exercise I was given while sitting in the wheelchair and with the leg rests off to the side, was to walk crab-like, one leg at a time moving myself forward without the use of any arms for assistance. At first, this procedure was very difficult, but again, with practice and patience the process became much easier. The benefit of performing this task was for the strengthening of my thighs. Eventually, under the guidance of a therapist, I was able to go outside to practice this maneuver and enjoy the nice summer weather. I know, learning these feats of skill may seem so elementary, however in my withered condition, these were new frontiers.

My ability to swallow still had not returned. The daily therapy sessions also included speech therapy. Having so many pieces of apparatus down my throat for so long and with the ever-present feeding tube down my nose and throat, and into my stomach, the swallow reflex was non-existent. The therapy was referred to as speech therapy, however, my speech had returned decently over the course of the last several weeks. What therapists concentrated on was trying to strengthen the throat muscles by having me perform a series of throat exercises with the hope of me eventually being able to swal-

low and enjoy food and liquid once again. I had two speech therapists that alternated with my training sessions. The tasks that I was
instructed to perform were; making the hard G and hard C sounds
in the back of my throat while forcing up air from the diaphragm. I
alternately repeated these "guh" and "kuh" sounds six or seven time
each. With making these series of goofy sounds throughout the day,
people passing by the room probably thought I was a nut case. Besides these exercises, there were other oral exercises that I was given
for strengthening the throat which resulted in even stranger sounds.
Thinking back on those throat exercises, I was probably very fortunate I didn't have a roommate. He or she would most likely have
jumped out of bed, trying to strangle me. I guess then, I wouldn't
have had to contend with those crazy throat exercises. The throat
exercises were performed with due diligence on my part for weeks
without any improvement. Weekly, I was taken in the wheelchair
by one of the speech therapists for a swallow test and each week
I failed. The test was a barium type x-ray for viewing my swallow
function. Of course, I couldn't even swallow the barium. I was offered an assortment of substances for my attempt at swallowing,
such as; pudding, Jell-O, apple sauce, and popsicle. While taking
a small portion of one of the items, a technician would x-ray my
throat during the attempted swallow process. The only problem was
the inability to swallow any of these treats. My reflex was to cough
up these substances, thus bringing the test to a halt for fear I might
aspirate. With the lungs already in a disadvantaged condition, they
didn't want to add any more problems. So it was back to my room
for more swallow exercises. It had been mentioned sometime earlier
about the removal of the feeding tube, however we were hesitant
because having the feeding tube implanted through the abdomen
might open up chances of more infection in my already compro-

mised body. We didn't feel there was a general consensus with doctors and nurses about the removal of the feeding tube. And also, we didn't feel they thought the feeding tube had much to do with my ability or lack thereof for swallowing. I don't think it was widely understood how the sensitivities of my connective tissue disorder affected the swallow reflex. However, after more discussion, we insisted they remove the feeding tube from my nose and throat. After all, nothing to this point had worked. The surgery to implant the G-Tube into my stomach needed to be approved by Dr. Oyer, who unfortunately was on vacation at the time. It meant we had to wait for his return before obtaining approval. "If it will help me pass the swallow test, let's do it!"

Again, I am mentioning, hospitals are not the proper environment for getting decent sleep. I thought, with exhaustion from "Boot Camp" during the day, I would have slept like a baby at night. The hallucinations I had experienced back in ICU reared their ugly heads once again. Only this time the hallucinations became a daytime event. I was laying in my bed looking out the window and saw a party going on with all my family, relatives, and friends outside in the courtyard. Even my parent's friends were all enjoying the party atmosphere with food and drinks in the lovely summer sun. I was so upset that I was not invited. How could they do this to me while I was stuck here in this darn bed? The entertainment for the afternoon was Randy Travis and his band. They pulled up in an old woody station wagon with an American flag hanging out the back and began setting up their equipment for the performance. However, after playing only one set they were asked to leave because their music was making so much noise it bothered many of the patients. So they loaded up and off they went. There had been a hotdog vendor outside during the afternoon celebration, and I wanted one of those great dogs all slathered in mustard. The problem was, I didn't have any money. I accused Mike, Mary, and my sisters of taking my money. "Why would you take my money? You know I love hotdogs!" Even in my hallucinatory state, I could see Mike and Mary looking at me and then at each other in total bewilderment thinking I had completely lost it. I am sure they both thought I was losing my mind. I also imagined friends coming in the room, then disappearing into the walls. I knew they were still there, and I felt comfort in knowing that, even though I couldn't see them. I envisioned Mary standing at the foot of my bed, dressed in a Swiss Bavarian costume, with her hair done in pigtails, then also vanishing into the wall. As my agitation increased during the course of that particular afternoon, Mary's frustration level increased to a breaking point, causing her to seek refuge back at the H.O.M.E. apartments. As the evening developed, I became more distressed over Mary's leaving, to the point of trying to get out of my bed and yelling at the nurses to call my wife. "I need my wife, I want my wife, please call my wife". "I am going to get out of this bed, call my wife!" "You stay in bed, Mr. Coover," one of the nurses yelled back from the nurses' station. As I remember back on those series of events, I am surprised men in white coats didn't show up with a straight jacket and tether me to the bed. Eventually, Mary came back and laid down next to me and with her presence I calmed down almost immediately. The next thing I remembered was waking up and being informed I had been asleep for almost a day. Wow, I certainly felt much better and all my demons seemed to have vanished. With the sedative I had been given, it was probably the best sleep I had experienced in months. Why didn't the hospital do that sooner? I was constantly asking for something to help with my sleep, however the sleep medications that had been previously administered just didn't do the trick. The psychiatric department did come by for a visit and an evaluation the following day. I told them that I felt fine and emphatically stated that all I needed was a good night's sleep. After their evaluation, they left in agreement.

Other concerns which were hindrances to my recovery in re-hab were constant urinary tract infections and high blood sugar. My blood sugar was tested twice a day with readings often over 100 which seemed rather strange because the only nutrition I consumed during that period came from the Nepro. However, Nepro being high in carbohydrates and protein might have been enough to drive up my numbers. A normal fasting reading should be around 80. Doctors and nurses even talked about the possibility of us purchasing a blood glucose testing kit when we returned home. I think my body just needed some time to become adjusted to all that had been thrown at it; new hearts, dialysis, rehab, and anti-rejection drugs, etc. Upon being released from the hospital and graduating to the H.O.M.E. apartments, the blood sugar concern was no longer an issue.

The throat exercises and the swallow tests continued until Dr. Oyer returned from his vacation to give approval for the implanta-tion of the feeding tube. So it was off to surgery for yet another procedure. Almost immediately after having the G-tube affixed and the removal of the bothersome nose/throat feeding tube, I miracu-lously began swallowing once again. Hurray! With the sensitivi-ties of my tissues due to the Ehlers-Danlos, having the feeding tube and the assortment of other paraphernalia down my throat for so many months, I strongly felt those obstacles were definite barriers to my ability for swallowing. The first recollection of being able to swallow was waking from sleep the first night after having the tube removed. I was thirsty and reached over to the table at the side of the bed grabbing a glass of water. Before realizing what I had done, I swallowed a big sip of water without choking. With my amazement, I buzzed the nurses' station, yelling that I had swallowed. After struggling for almost four months, I was more than elated. It was certainly a moment for celebration even though it was the middle of the night. I wished the permanent removal of the nose/throat tube had occurred weeks earlier. Possibly my swallow reflex would have returned much sooner. Upon hearing I had swallowed, the hospital scheduled me for another swallow test on August 15. I felt with this seventh attempt I would be successful. I passed! I finally passed!

In between therapy sessions and on weekends when I didn't have much formal therapy, I appreciated telephone conversations and visits with friends. Audrey, Steve, Lisa, Paul, and Vern and Kay from my work came for visits. An old high school classmate and friend, Tom, stopped by one evening reminiscing as to where all the years had gone. Friends Jay and Casey, Steve and Helaine, and our former neighbors, DiAnn and Terry also took time from their schedules for much appreciated visits. Denny, who I had known for years and had called Mary a couple of times to check up on my progress, stopped by for an enjoyable afternoon visit. She was the real estate agent who had handled the sale of my mother's house the previous year.

Another issue I had to conquer before being released from the hospital was learning to use the bathroom by myself. Sliding from the wheelchair on to the toilet and then trying to get back into the wheelchair was almost impossible for me. Proper leg, back, and arm strength was something I still hadn't obtained. However, after numerous attempts and with the help of a great nurse, Chris, I was able to be marginally successful.

14
Seeing Some Progress

Mary

On Thursday, July 6, my friends Rosie and Marylou came to cheer me up. We had such a great time playing games and staying up talking until late in the evening. Unfortunately, they had to drive back to Santa Rosa early on Friday. I took Don to the atrium about 12:30 for his first Bing concert. Then Don had dialysis, which was scheduled from 1:30 to 5:00. While he was there, Christine Hartley came to tell him they were moving him to rehab later that day. So about 8:00 that evening he was transferred to C-1, room 101. It was not a smooth transition. I had called Michael to tell him the new phone number, but when he tried to call Don, the call wouldn't go through because rehab didn't allow calls after 8:00 p.m. Then Don's new nurse wanted a list of all his drugs and their dosage. Of course we tried to explain that the list was in our red binder and we didn't have it anymore. Intermediate had taken it away from us.

All this agitated Don and he started complaining that he felt he was in prison. If he only knew that this was only the beginning and that he would later understand why they called rehab, "Boot Camp."

The occupational therapist came in early on Saturday with some gadgets to help Don dress himself. One was a grabber to pull on his sweat pants up over his rear end while sitting in the wheelchair. Then there was a plastic sleeve to pull his socks up and a metal rod to slip his shoes on. Tara, Spencer, and the children arrived at the hospital about 12:30. Don had P.T. for an hour, speech for an hour, and then he was so tired he slept until 5:00. When I came back after dinner we played dominos until 8:00. His spirits were pretty good, but little things still agitated him. They were still asking for his list of drugs, which they should have had and we didn't. We found out later that they had removed some of the information from his binder they thought wasn't needed anymore and sent it to Records in the basement.

Audrey and Steve from Don's work came in the morning of July 9. Don's sister Candi, her husband Dan, and their daughter Lauren came for an hour in the early afternoon. But the most exciting thing that happened that day was Don's first shower. Up until this point, he had only sponge baths. Larry, one of the male nurses took Don down the hall to a special shower that had a large plastic seat. Larry lifted him out of the wheelchair an onto this seat which had raised arms for support. Although I wasn't in the room with them, Don later told me he did most of the work himself; using the bar of soap and washcloth while the shower gently rinsed over him. I am sure Larry had to help him dry off, get dressed, and get back into the wheelchair, but Don exited the shower room with a huge smile on his face.

The next day being a Monday and the first day of the week turned out to be his first full day of therapy and dialysis together. He had physical therapy from 10:00 to 11:00, occupational therapy from 11:00 to 12:00, and speech therapy from 2:00 to 3:00. He ended up having dialysis that day from 3:00 to 7:00 which was longer than usual because it was necessary to stop part way through. Accidently, his feeding tube had not been turned off and the Nepro was still flowing for a while before someone noticed. This caused Don to become nauseated until they figured out the problem. To make matters worse, he had accidently been given a stool softener causing an attack of diarrhea. The poor guy was worn out by the time they got him back to his room. I changed his diaper, but he barely had enough energy to roll from side to side for me to clean him. It was a major undertaking every time Don was cleaned up. It was necessary for someone to push him on to his side because he didn't have enough strength himself. Then with the little strength he had in his arms, he held on to the railings on the side of the bed while we washed him, changed his diaper, and sometimes his bed linens. Unfortunately, this occurrence seemed to repeat itself quite frequently. That day he had messed his clothes, so I took them back to the apartment to be washed. Luckily, I had just bought him a second set of exercise clothes.   The doctors also informed us that day, the surgery for the permanent catheter in his arm for dialysis would have to be put off until Don was finished with rehab because of the insurance.

It's bad enough when one person is cranky, but on Tuesday, I awoke with a sore throat putting me in a rotten mood. When I arrived at Don's room and saw that he was tired and irritable, I should have turned around and gone back to bed. It turned out that they had bumped up his speech time and he wasn't dressed yet. He was trying to dress himself each day, but it still took a long time. At 9:30 he had O.T. for half an hour. Regrettably he was so tired from getting dressed that he made everyone else's day a living hell. He did have a productive session with Ryan in P.T., but had to leave early to be cleaned up by me again. He was still having numerous accidents because of the Nepro and stool softeners. When we did get him back to the gym with Ryan, he amazed us by standing up at the parallel bars almost completely by himself. I told him it was the new outfit with the t-shirt from Tara that said, "World's Greatest Grandpa."

They had to pick Don up early the next day for his heart biopsy. This effected his therapy schedule, which in turn effected Don's mood. He didn't do well with change and especially sudden change. By the time he came back from the biopsy, he was sore, tired, and irritable because they had trouble getting the line from his neck down to his heart. Because of Don's connective tissue disorder, this would be a common problem during many of his biopsies. The biopsy was in the morning, so he didn't have any therapy that day. I was disappointed that they couldn't fit in at least one half hour for recreational therapy. I felt it was one thing that relaxed Don. One nice thing that happened that day was the promptness of taking him to dialysis. He was scheduled for 2:30. They were in his room at exactly 2:30 for transport and he was hooked up to the machine by 3:00. He was finished with the session by 6:15. Everything was going so well, then the other shoe fell. Poor Don had to wait until 7:45 for the transport to take him back to his room. The other bad news that day was his weigh-in for dialysis showed he had lost weight, which he could not afford. He was down to 104.6 pounds. His nurse was a trainee that day who was having numerous problems. First, she gave him his anti-fungus medicine for his mouth into his I.V. We had to point this out to her. Next, she took forty minutes to change his diaper, which I had to change again because it was still a mess. Lastly, she tried very hard, but she was as slow as molasses and dropped a syringe on the dirty floor and was going to use it for an injection into the I.V. before we stopped her. Don was so happy when they posted the next day's schedule on the bulletin board that night. He had the nurse he liked and P.T. with Ryan the first thing in the morning. We both loved Ryan and Don was excited about standing by himself and trying to take a step using the parallel bars. Just before I left him that evening, the speech therapist came in to say they would be waiting one or two more weeks before giving him his next swallow test.

Don had another rough day on July, 13. He woke up grumpy and it never got better. First, they changed his schedule again. Then the doctors came in to strongly recommend having a feeding tube surgically implanted in his stomach. Don was vehement about waiting and talking to Dr. Oyer regarding any more surgeries. However, Dr. Oyer was in Europe for two more weeks. Don dosed off at 7:30 that night, which was my clue to leave.

My goodness! What a great day he had on Friday! He was in a super mood all day. Everything flowed perfectly. He did miss his respiratory therapy because of his dialysis, but they were able to fit in a session of recreational therapy which was a huge plus. Don and I played dominos and his spirits were boosted because he won. His attention span wasn't great, but games got his mind off his health. It also cheered him up that he had a visit from Vern and Kay, two friends of Don's, who were in their eighties, yet drove all the way down from Petaluma to see Don. I think they were both taken aback to see how thin and weak Don was. However, their visit meant the world to both Don and me.

He took his first four steps on the parallel bars on Saturday, July 15, with a little help from the physical therapist. Don was so excited about these first few steps, but at the same time, began talking about a feeding tube in his stomach being less cumbersome than a tube hanging out of his nose which got in his way during physical therapy. That night, nurses tried giving him a cherry popsicle. He didn't swallow, just tasted and spit it out. He loved that cherry popsicle, something cold and delicious. He had satisfaction written all over his face.

I didn't get a lot of sleep on Saturday night, because the smoke alarm in the apartments went off for a fourth time since I had moved in. It seems there are worse cooks in the world than me and why would anyone be cooking in the middle of the night anyway? Even though I was probably not in prime form, we had a visit from our friends, Jay and Casey, who were shocked at how thin Don was. Then DiAnn and Terry came in the afternoon and said over and over how great he looked. Unfortunately, DiAnn had entered the room carrying a soda cup that Don immediately zeroed in on and it held his salivating attention throughout their visit. It was wonderful to have DiAnn, who was a nurse, explain all the medical things to us such as the different options Don had for dialysis when he was released from the hospital to go home.

Monday was a long, hard day for Don. He tried to stand with the walker by the sink to self-catheterize, but got less than 50cc. Then, just as he was about to leave for O.T. at 10:00, a nurse came in to say he had an infection in his urine and everyone who entered his room was to wear yellow paper gowns, masks, paper booties, and gloves. No one was to touch Don without the garb. Next, his dialysis was postponed until after 5:00 that night and they would have to do it in his room because of the infectious disease. That meant bringing all the heavy machinery into his room and extra time for setup. Lastly, his weight that day plummeted to 102.8 pounds.

Four doctors from infectious disease came to see us about 5:00 p.m. on July 18. We were told an antibiotic would be started on Don sometime soon. Then Christine Hartley came in with great news that Dr. Oyer would be returning in two days. At that time, we could all discuss Don's swallowing or lack thereof. They were talking about giving him another swallow test the following week on Tuesday. If he didn't pass, they would be putting the new feeding tube in his stomach. It was funny about people coming into his room, some people put all the paper precaution wear on before entering and some didn't put anything on. I didn't wear any because I felt I was already exposed and the fact that I was in his room all day wasn't going to be altered by some paper gowns. We never knew if it was to protect Don from the exposure of people coming in or for their protection from Don.

Don was finally seeing some progress since he had been in re-hab. Wednesday was an upbeat day for him. He had P.T. and O.T. in the morning. Then I took him to the recreation room where he got on the computer and deleted quite a few of our old e-mails. We both felt so good about cleaning up our inbox. In dialysis that day, they only took off .5 liters, so Don wasn't as sick to his stomach as he became when they took off more. While having his dialysis, two urologists came in to say his prostrate was just fine. This was great news because I don't think he could have handled anything else going wrong.

On Thursday, July 20, Don had a super day in P.T. with Ryan. I'm just sorry I wasn't around to see it, but he walked with his walk-er all the way across the P.T. room with no assistance. He was so excited and when I got to him he made me promise to write it in my journal that night. I had to drive back to Santa Rosa that day, however he did have visits from our friends Denny, Helaine, and her husband, Steve. Don shared his good news with them.

Don got discouraged so easily. And because he had to have Ryan's help with walking the last couple of feet down the hallway, Don felt he had somehow failed. On Friday the speech therapist said he couldn't have the feeding tube removed from his nose before the swallow test, so he felt sure of failing the test again. The case worker said that they were hoping to discharge Don on August 8. She would give us a copy of the goals he was supposed to have accomplished by then. One of the top goals was to be eating. We think there was something wrong with their scales though because when she weighed him it said 112.5 pounds. That meant he had gained almost 9 pounds in four days since they had weighed him in dialysis. We think one of the weights was way off.

Saturday, July 22 was another day of schedule changes, but Don did so well. They were able to fit his P.T., O.T., and speech all in between a visit from our friends DiAnn and Terry. I was so thrilled to see Don accomplish everything the therapist asked of him because the weather had turned extremely hot. Not only was his room not air conditioned, but the heater got stuck in the on position with the outside temperature way over 100 degrees. Don never complained once. I wish I could say I didn't either. Sunday, Monday, and Tuesday were all 105 degrees or hotter. I thought we had it bad, but the air conditioning also went out for parts of the hospital, including the cafeteria and kitchen which meant the kitchen staff had to work in sweltering heat for over two days.

On Wednesday, July 26, Don failed another swallow test, meaning the next step was putting the "plug," (the stomach feeding tube), surgically in and taking out the one in his nose. Don was upset about another surgery, but at the same time, realistic that it was for the best. We were also hoping that it might even help his nausea and maybe the swelling he was still having in his feet and ankles. His white blood count was low so they had to adjust his feedings, his antibiotics, and his amount of dialysis out take.

On Friday, they only took off 150 cc during dialysis so Don's feet were still quite swollen. That made it harder for Don to use his walker. At this time, Don was using the walker more and more to try to get around by himself. His arms were beginning to have more strength. And although his legs and arms were as skinny as twigs, his ability to use them was increasing every day. We noticed a huge improvement in his physical abilities as a result of the therapy in the rehab unit.

Because the smoke alarm in the apartments went off again Friday night, I got very little sleep. Don called me early Saturday morning begging me to get right over to the hospital. When I got there at about 8:30, the nurse pulled me aside to tell me that Don had had a terrible night hallucinating, trying to get out of the bed, and shouting for me. He hadn't had a lot of sleep the previous few nights and the lack of sleep had caught up with him. These were some of the worst days I had had with him since going to Stanford. He looked like he was swatting bees away and he would ask weird questions like, "Did I get the T-bones ready? Are the desserts ready to take to Mom's? Did I talk to Norm who was just around the corner?" At one point Don thought I was wearing lederhosen and had my hair in braids. I told him I didn't care how he pictured me as long as he pictured me thin. It got to the point I couldn't stand seeing Don like that, so I left about 8:00 that night pleading with the nurses to give him something to help him sleep.

* * * *

They gave him two doses of sleep medication and he still didn't sleep through the night. So on Sunday, July 30, after five nights of no sleep, our children had to him talking to the walls and carrying on that there was a conspiracy against him. He thought a dog was jumping on the bed, he thought a friend came to the hospital but wouldn't talk to him, and he was sure a hotdog man was just outside his window, but I had stolen all his money so he couldn't buy a hotdog. Don was positive that Randy Travis was performing somewhere and I wouldn't take him to see him. He was also positive that important papers from his work had been dropped off and I threw them away. Then he started to cry because everyone was against him. Joel, his nurse asked me to stay the night with him. The doctors were to give him an anti-hallucinate drug and a relaxation medication. I stayed until about 11:00 p.m., but he never stopped talking and thrashing in his bed, so I left to get some much needed sleep for myself. I had tried sleeping next to Don in his little bed but that was ridiculous. I left telling the nurses that I was no help and they were on their own getting him to sleep.

When I arrived at Don's rehab room on Monday, July 31, it was about 8:00 a.m. and he was sound asleep. The nurse told me they had given him a sleeping pill and an anti-hallucinate drug about midnight, but they had no effect on Don. So at 4:00 a.m. they gave him another dose. By 5:00 a.m. he was sound asleep and slept through until 2:30 in the afternoon. They actually had to wake him up for his 3:00 dialysis.

After working in my classroom all day on August 1, to get set up for the new school year, I drove back to Palo Alto just as Don was finishing his speech therapy about 4:00. He said he had fallen while working with Ryan. However, no huge bruises, and it was a great workout. Since Don had been on the prednisone as one of his anti-rejection meds and because of his Ehlers-Danlos Syndrome, we had seen quite a few bruises on him; something we would need to watch for the rest of his life. Don also had a great O.T. session that day. He practiced getting from his wheelchair to the toilet. He still wasn't able to get his pants pulled down, however getting himself to the bathroom was a huge step in the right direction. The p.m. nurse showed me how to administer his meds in his I.V. line and how to give the feedings when he got his "plug." It was just fine with me because I wasn't feeling comfortable about moving Don to the apartments and me being his sole support for all his medical needs.

Don had a full and very productive day on Wednesday. He walked the whole length of the hallway using his walker and only two stops to sit and rest in the wheelchair. Ryan was just as impressed as I was. Don worked on the computer for recreational therapy for half an hour that day. Next, he had O.T. for an hour and then another hour of P.T. in the afternoon before dialysis. To top it all off, he had a new pic line put in from 12:00 to 1:15 while I was listening to the music concert in the atrium. Although he wasn't eating as yet and he couldn't walk by himself, he was doing so much better than just a few weeks before.

For O.T. on Thursday, Julie took him to a special bathroom where she taught him how to get in and out of the bathroom using a plastic seat that fit across the tub. He would get himself out of the wheelchair using the walker, then swing around to sit on a special tub seat. Then he would twist himself around pulling one leg at a time over the edge of the tub. That afternoon, Ryan and his assistant walked us over to the apartments for an introduction to functioning on our own. I was petrified! Ryan had Don try things like getting in and out of bed, the chair and couch in the living room, and maneuvering the wheelchair around corners. Another thing Ryan had Don try was sitting on the toilet and getting back up by himself. Since Don had no real leg muscles, it was next to impossible. So the next thing on my list to purchase was going to be a five inch toilet seat riser. When I was behind Don with his walker going from the bathroom back to the bedroom, Don fell and it took Ryan and me together to get him back up. I was scared stiff of not being able to help Don once he was discharged from the hospital. He was to continue with therapy, but it was going to be just me taking care of him, and me alone.

August 4, was a great day for Don and a super day for me. My friends Donna, Lorol, and Janet came to stay with me for the night on their way to shopping in San Francisco. They dropped off their things at the apartment, then we all walked over to see Don who was thrilled to see them. Then when we arrived back to the apartments, I started to take the stairs rather than the elevator. It was only one flight and I always took the stairs for exercise. As we started to walk up, Lorol turned and said, "You know Mary it's not safe alone in a stairway. Someone could attack you." I don't remember laughing that hard since I got to Stanford. I looked at her and said, "Honey, if someone wanted to attack me here, I would have to get them out of the wheelchair, hold them up, and do all the work myself." Almost everyone in the building were patients recovering from transplant surgery. We had such a great time laughing the whole night. Lorol and I sat up on the blow up mattress talking until past midnight. It was a godsend having a break from my worries about Don.

Don was very upset with me when I arrived about 8:30 a.m. after my friends left on Saturday. He hadn't slept well and the morning only got worse when I had him on the bedpan right when O.T. came for his therapy. To make matters worse, he hadn't received his 8:00 a.m. meds. It was now 9:00, and he wouldn't be returning from therapy until way after 10:00 a.m. He was so angry, he threw the bedpan against the wall. All I could say was, "Good arm strength." Needless to say, we changed his O.T. to the afternoon, when he would hopefully be in a better mood. He did very well in P.T. and O.T. even though he grumbled the whole time that he was too tired and they were working him too hard. If Don only knew, I kept telling his therapist that he needed to be pushed.

On Sunday, Don was in a great mood. There were a couple of reasons. First he slept for eight hours during the night. Next, he watched golf and the Giants, who finally won against the Rockies. Lastly, he was able to get out of bed and to the walker all by himself. Granted, the bed was as high as possible, but he slid his legs over the side and got to a standing position without any assistance. We were both so pleased that I wanted to shout down the halls. But controlling myself, we had Don walk the whole hallway with me following behind pushing the wheelchair. Since Don was already garbed up in his yellow paper gear from head to toe, I checked him out of the hospital for the afternoon so we could spend it together at the apartment. He watched a little football, (we only got three stations on the TV.) Then I took him back for his 6:00 meds and much needed sleep before his feeding tube surgery scheduled for the next morning.

On Monday, August 7, someone from surgery came to tell Don they would be taking him early to the surgery room. So of course, we told O.T. and P.T. that we needed to reschedule. We waited, and waited, and waited. Murphy's Law of hurry up and wait. They finally took him shortly after 10:00, saying it would be about a half hour surgery. At 11:30 I asked the surgery receptionist if she could find out what was taking so long. The good news was that he was doing just fine. The bad news was that he had just come out of surgery and would be kept in recovery quite a while. When he did get back to the room, he was groggy and complaining of his painful incision. He had been given morphine and because he was out of it, I left at 7:30. On my way out, I ran into Alice, one of the pink ladies from surgery floor 2, who was thrilled to hear how well Don was doing. She was one of my support group who helped me through the first six weeks of Don's stay in ICU. She told me that she continued to tell everyone of Don's miraculous recovery. And to me, he truly was a miracle.

On Tuesday morning, Don was in a lot of pain so they gave him Vicodin which helped quite a bit. However, even with less pain, he wasn't in the mood for physical therapy. He had O.T. both in the morning and in the afternoon where they had him working on molding putty in his hands. I was a little surprised for two reasons that the speech therapist tried having him swallow orange juice that day. The first reason was that Don was still having trouble swallowing and secondly because orange juice is high in potassium which Don's failing kidneys had trouble processing. Watching all those issues worried me once we got Don to the apartment. Christine Hartley and Evelyn the social worker came to Don's room to answer questions in regards to his discharge and to give a formal teaching lesson on his meds, feedings, appointments, and who to call for future questions.

On Wednesday and Thursday Don was still in pain and still asking for Vicodin. In the afternoon, Don had a massage and a visit by the doctors who informed us that Don would be wearing the lovely paper gowns until he was discharged. Then early in the evening, the pharmacist from the hospital came to watch me administer Don's drugs and make sure I could do it once we got to the apartment.

They were all fairly self-explanatory although we were taken aback to learn they were $173 each month. This was only to be a part of the meds that Don would be needing. Friday, August 11, was a busy day for Don. He had a heart biopsy, P.T., O.T., and dialysis. That evening they also started his bolus feeding in his stomach "plug." His stomach was sore yet from the surgery, but he was so happy to finally have the tube out of his nose.

The next day I brought some low sodium beef broth, Sprite, and a bottled water to try having him take liquids by the mouth. He did alright, but we were anxious to get him to the apartment where we could monitor his feedings and the medication on our own schedule. Sometimes the nurses were really busy so they would show up two hours late for his medication times. That in turn would throw off his four feedings every six hours. Then we had to wait two hours after his anti-rejection medication (Gengraf) before he could have any foods. He was given 360 cc of food and 150 cc of water every six hours which did two things: filled him up to bloating and gave him the runs, (so much fun to clean up.) His diapers never did hold everything, so it meant changing his clothes and sheets a couple of times a day.

Sunday and Monday passed with very little change other than Tara Anne coming to see Don while I was up in Santa Rosa getting my classroom ready for the new school year. She brought a beautiful homemade anniversary banner for the apartment because Wednesday was going to be our twentieth wedding anniversary. Don called me on Tuesday, August 15, while I was at school to tell me he had FINALLY passed the swallow test. We had been saying for weeks and weeks, once he got that blasted feeding tube out of his nose and throat, he would be able to swallow. And sure enough that is exactly what happened.

I taught school all day with the long term substitute on Wednesday, August 16, then drove back just as Candi and Ardi were leaving after spending a few hours midday with Don. They had taken him to the music concert in the atrium which featured Dr. Lawrence Mathers, the doctor who had cheered me up with his beautiful music during the first couple of months I had been at Stanford.

Don had P.T. that morning where they gave him a new walker, a children's wheelchair, and a toilet commode that we would take over to the apartment. I gave Don some anniversary presents: a collapsible walking cane, a mortar & pestle to grind his pills, and a relaxation CD. He gave me a beautiful card that Tara Anne had purchased for him when she visited on Monday. I had planned on spending the night with Don in the hospital room after having a delicious hospital dinner, UGH, but they couldn't find a lounge chair for me to be brought into the room for sleeping.

15
Moving to the Apartments

Don

August 17, was a milestone day! It was the first day I consumed actual chewable food since the end of April. That morning I was wheeled down to a commons room at the end of the rehab corridor for a breakfast of pancakes, eggs, sausage, fruit, juice, and tea. I was overjoyed that I was having a real meal after being on a liquid diet through my nose for so many months. Surprisingly, there were no issues with swallowing and my appetite was actually very good. Now, I was on the right track towards a full recovery. Up to this point, I felt as though I had been treading water and not making much progress. Hallelujah! All at once things got kicked into high gear. Maybe it was the result of celebrating our twentieth anniversary the day before in my room. I enjoyed a cup of broth as Mary dined on a meal from the cafeteria. The stars must have been properly aligned for what was to happen the afternoon of the 17th. After so many agonizing months, I was released from

Stanford as an in-house patient! We gathered up all my gear and medicines for the one block wheelchair ride over to the H.O.M.E. Apartments for my continuing recovery.

Sometime earlier, Ryan from rehab had taken us over to the apartment for my introductory tour, showing me how to navigate with my wheelchair and walker through the living room, bedroom, bathroom, and kitchen. The apartment wasn't that big, maybe four hundred square feet, so the lesson didn't take that long. We were instructed not to have any area rugs on the floor which could create hazards for my newly acquired, although feeble walking ability. I was assigned a nurse for weekly visits and a physical therapist for every other day training. Mary found a high-boy seat for the toilet at a local drug store and our friend, Donna had given us a bench for me to sit on while taking a shower. My strength was still way below par so those devices were great aids for helping with my daily duties. I found that I became fairly proficient at piloting the walker around the apartment. Whenever I was in bed, sitting in a chair, on the toilet, or in the shower, the walker was my best friend, always in front of or right next to me. The wheelchair was now only used for our trips to the hospital or for any excursions outside the apartments.

When released from the hospital, I still had the G-tube in my stomach for which Mary had to use for administering many of the anti-rejection drugs; Gengraf, Cellcept, etc. and drugs for fighting pneumonia and infections; Bactrim and Valcyte. Mary had stopped by the Plaza Pharmacy across from the apartments, picking up a box full of prescriptions. We even brought a case of the lovely Nepro with us from the hospital. A binder had been provided to us, listing all the drugs and vitamins with instructions as to their usage and time of day for administering. At one point, the list was as many as twenty items. Prior to the transplant, I had read accountings of other heart transplant patients who were sent home with a toolbox full of medicines. The image always bothered me, thinking I would have to carry a box full of prescriptions around with me for the rest of my life. So when I saw all the medicines lined up on the kitchen counter in the apartment, I freaked out. Seeing how well I had adjusted to my oral intake of real food and with no problem swallowing, the G-tube was removed during one of my check-up visits at the hospital, less than two weeks after going to the apartments. I was now mostly free of external attachments. The only one remaining was the neck catheter used for dialysis treatments.

The apartments, being so close in proximity to the hospital, became very convenient for our daily trips back and forth for various clinic appointments and dialysis treatments. Mary would wheel me to my every other day dialysis which were most usually on Mondays, Wednesdays, and Fridays. The dialysis room was on the ground level of the hospital, past the atrium, and down near the cancer wing of the hospital. Now, with me being treated as an outpatient, dialysis treatments seemed to be much more bearable. I wasn't as agitated with the process and my bouts of nausea and vomiting were less frequent. I could get out of the wheelchair unassisted, step over onto the scale, and then walk the few steps, again without help, over to the dialysis chair. I knew in three to four hours, I would be up and out of there, on my way back to the apartments.

Not too long after joining Mary at the apartment, I was trying out my navigational skills with the walker and fell going between the bathroom and the living room. I tripped over one of the area rugs Mary had bought to dress up the apartment. We knew immediately why we had been instructed not to have any loose rugs on the floor. I guess we had to learn the hard way. Although, the rug probably afforded some cushioning between my bony body and the hard lino-leum. After landing in a clump on the floor and realizing I couldn't get up, we both panicked as to how to fix my predicament. Mary tried to no avail. We then had an idea there might be someone in an adjoining apartment that could assist. Most of the other patients in the building were no better off than me. However, a strong care giver might be the answer. Finally, after being gone for a while, Mary returned with a big football player type guy who scooped me up and plunked me back into the wheelchair.

I enjoyed the every other day visits from Barbara the physical therapist. However, her one hour visits continued in the same challenging style as I had experienced at the hospital. But, I guess that was the intended purpose. No pain no gain! If I was ever to get back to anything close to where I was before, I had a long way yet to go. Our first sessions involved a wheelchair ride to the hallway outside our apartment door. The hallway had a vestibule with a four foot high railing. Barbara instructed me to hold on to the railing, at the same time taking sideway steps in one direction and then back in the other direction. The distance of the railing was approximately thirty feet, so negotiating the sixty foot distance with this newly prescribed movement was quite taxing. I progressed on to walking the length of our second floor hallway down and back with the use of the walker. As I became more adept with my assignments, we started taking wheelchair rides out to the front of the apartment building where I would push the wheelchair in front of me while walking behind, very much the same as I had done in rehab at the hospital. Mary and Barbara would walk on each side of me for guidance and protection as I walked slowly trying to negotiate the bumpy and somewhat uneven tree lined sidewalk. Our trip took us past the front of the apartments to a medical building next door where we would turn around for the trip back. I was still wobbly and not very sure footed, but each time we practiced I felt stronger and more accomplished.

The next event in my training was to relearn walking stairs. Barbara would wheel me to the elevator for a ride to the first floor of the apartments where we would go to the stairwell for my attempt at walking back up to the second floor. Other than learning to stand, the stair sessions were probably the second most difficult and physically demanding activity I had undertaken to this point. My first go at this task was with Barbara holding me under the arm on my right side while I grabbed the railing for dear life with my left hand. Having the strength in my stick legs for supporting my body, one leg at a time, one step at a time, was next to impossible. I found it difficult enough standing on two legs, never mind shifting total body weight from one leg to the other. Again, after several weeks of practice, my strength and ability returned to where I could come to terms with the stairs. Although, I navigated cautiously with a cane in one hand and holding on to the railing with the other, I eventually advanced to walking the wheelchair ramp up to the apartment entrance. I had a choice of two canes. Mary had bought me a collapsible one which was very light and stored easily in the back pocket of the wheelchair or in her purse. The other was very unique, to say the least. On one of Mary's trips to Santa Rosa, a long narrow box was waiting on our front porch. Much to her surprise, inside was a three foot cane made from the reproductive organ of a bull. It was quite heavy, gnarled, and finished with a shiny coat of resin. It had been sent to me from Mary's nephew, John Meyer, Jr. who lives in Wisconsin. What a great gift! Even to this day the cane makes for a great show and tell conversation piece. That must have been some bull!!

Mary and I settled into a decent routine during our stay in the apartment. My appetite remained good and no issues reoccurred with swallowing. (That damn feeding tube.) However, my weight gain was almost non-existent. Mary had purchased a scale to track my weight. I was almost afraid to stand on it. After several weeks at the apartment, I was lucky if I weighed 110 - 112 pounds. Historically, my weight had always been between 155 - 160 pounds; even up to the last several months before the transplant. At the current rate, it would be years until I approached a decent body weight once again. Considering the distress my body had recently experienced, and attempting to get through the recovery period while contending with a bladder condition and kidney failure was almost over burdensome. My kidney function hadn't returned as hoped. The good news was, I had a great, new, and well-functioning heart. However, the bad news was I was now headed for years of dialysis treatments while waiting for a kidney transplant.

I continued with the every other day dialysis treatments and once a week visits for heart clinic appointments and blood testing. Our mode of transportation was usually by wheelchair since it was much quicker. I think we knew every crack, bump, weed, and piece of gum on the sidewalk between the apartments and the hospital. Before I was capable of walking, and relying only on the wheelchair as my mode of transportation, I was provided a new appreciation of how difficult it must be for people who are confined for years in a wheelchair. At one point in the rehabilitation process, I thought moving around by wheelchair might be the best I could ever expect.

Once again, I became adept at performing the required intermittent catheterization process. I usually performed it two to three times daily, every day. The color and consistency of the urine had returned to what could be considered fairly normal. However, the volume produced was very limited. Urinary tract infections continued in the same manner as had been the issue at the hospital. Antibiotics would clear up the problem in the short term. But, a week later I might have another infection. Of course, the culprit, was the combination of anti-rejection drugs and the catheter process. We knew anti-rejection drugs interfered with the body's immune system. So adding the catheter procedure to the mix, which we had learned years previously, adds chances of introducing bacteria into the body, I was now facing a double whammy; an immune suppressed body and that body trying to fight off infection. Like trying to roll a rock up a hill, it's almost a losing battle.

Transplant patients have to be diligent in their approach with taking anti-rejection drugs. If I had to pass along one piece of information, it would be to remain true to your schedule of taking medications. In my situation, it was every twelve hours; 10:00 a.m. and 10:00 p.m. Proper blood levels of anti-rejection drugs are needed to remain consistent for fighting rejection. In occasional discussions with other heart transplant patients and upon hearing they had experienced situations of some rejection because they weren't as well disciplined as they should have been, I knew if I was ever to have any rejection, it wouldn't be from not taking my scheduled drugs. In fact, I am probably too anal about it.

One afternoon Mary and I were involved in a round table discussion with other heart transplant recipients, patients waiting for a transplant, and their family members or care givers. The discussion was moderated by Mary Burge who we felt comfortable with since we had interacted with her on several previous occasions. The gathering was held in the same building where we had our first meeting with Dr. Oyer some two years earlier. There was a variety of people in different stages of recovery and some were there to obtain information on their awaiting transplant. We told stories of our individual situations which put us all at ease and provided a camaraderie knowing we weren't alone in our paths to a better life. At the meeting, we met a couple from Hawaii who had moved to the Palo Alto area to be closer to Stanford while the husband was waiting for a new heart. He had been an airline mechanic for a major airline and had been on the transplant list for almost a year. As his health declined, they were quite concerned with how much longer he might have to wait. His long wait was due largely to having an O Positive blood type.

I became less dependent on the wheelchair and the walker and was able to move more independently with only using the cane for short distances. Mary and I ventured around the Stanford and Palo Alto area with taking trips to church, museums, and the occasional lunch or dinner. Our next door neighbors in Santa Rosa, Bill and Gloria, drove down and treated us to a nice lunch at a restaurant on University Avenue in Palo Alto. These events were almost as if they were first time experiences for me. It was wonderful becoming part of the real world once again. We even ventured to P.F. Changs where, yes, I enjoyed one of their ice cold lemonades. My prayers were answered! It's funny how the simplest things can mean so much.

There is a Rodin collection at the Cantor Arts Center on the Stanford campus. I didn't know up until that time that it even existed there. Mary had discovered it on one of her outings while I was still in intensive care. As a treat, Mary wheeled me over in the wheelchair since it was quite a distance from the apartments. It turned out to be one of our longest outings. We went on a weekend when I didn't have any dialysis or scheduled therapy. The collection of Rodin bronzes is one of the largest collections in the world. It was something I will long remember.

On one of our outings, we decided to take in an afternoon movie at the Stanford Theater on University Avenue in downtown Palo Alto. University Avenue is a quaint tree lined street with many upscale shops, restaurants and sidewalk cafes. The theater was an old time movie house; unlike the multiplex theaters we have today. Mary dropped me off in front and went on to park the car. With cane in hand, I started walking toward the box office to purchase our tickets. Without being cognizant of the six inch curb I was about to approach, and not in proper position to coordinate my step/cane function, I fell down on the curb between two diagonally parked cars. I was so elated that I could be independent enough for venturing about on my own that I neglected to notice the approaching curb. I sat there in the gutter trying to get back up to no avail. Sitting that low to the ground and grabbing on to a bumper of one of the cars, I still didn't have enough strength in my legs to get up. I started to panic. I told Mary I would be waiting right in front of the box office. If she didn't see me waiting, I knew she would think something terrible had happened. I knew somehow I had to get out of my predicament. I shouted over to the box office attendant and to people walking by on the sidewalk if they would help me up. I must have sat there for five minutes being completely ignored. Even seeing that I was struggling, no one stopped for assistance. It certainly speaks volumes in regards to today's society. People just don't want to get involved. After all, a sixty-one year old man sitting in the gutter might have hit someone over the head with his cane and taken their money.

My recovery had advanced to the point where some of our outings allowed us to adventure outside the Stanford/Palo Alto area. We took an afternoon trip to Half Moon Bay, on the coast, about a thirty minute drive from our apartment. Another time, I rode with Mary to our home in Santa Rosa to check on a couple of weeks of accumulated mail. On a Friday, after one of my dialysis treatments, we journeyed up to our cabin in the Tahoe area for a weekend getaway. I didn't have to be back for my next treatment until Monday morning. Of course, Mary handled all the driving. How thrilling it was to be a participant in activities that I questioned if I would ever have the ability to enjoy again.

In September, Mary had an opportunity to attend her fortieth high school reunion in Minnesota, but I wasn't to the point in my recovery where I could be left alone. So we made arrangements where my sisters and my son Mike would share the duty. I managed to arrange reservations for Mary's trip on our laptop in the social room of the apartments. The social room was the only place in the building for picking up a decent internet signal. Mary flew out of San Jose International Airport early on a Friday morning and was to return Sunday evening. My sisters stayed with me during the day on Friday and were relieved of their duty with Mike's arrival later in the afternoon. Mike stayed with me Saturday night and the next day drove us down for a visit in Santa Cruz, where he lived. After bringing me back to the apartment later in the afternoon, I waited for Mary's return that evening. She had a wonderful time seeing fellow classmates and nuns, most of which she hadn't seen since she graduated. It was a nice get away and a much needed change of pace for her. Mary's life the past several months was only about dealing with me. Worrying if I was going to survive, dealing with doctors and nurses, signing authorizations for my many procedures, being my advocate, and catering to my many needs, was a 24/7 project. When she wasn't at the hospital, she was tending to issues at her school and taking care of our personal finances. Mary was a real trooper considering what I had put her through. She always remained positive and never wavered from her upbeat and bubbly personality. I am sure she was hurting on the inside, but it rarely showed on the outside. Mary is my candidate to receive the award for the world's best wife.

All the months of lying in a hospital bed at Stanford and even after moving to the apartments, we witnessed a constant whirr of helicopter traffic landing and taking off from the hospitals' helipad which was situated on the roof of the hospital. On each occasion, we imagined another organ being transported with its team of doctors ready and waiting for the transplant.

As a heart transplant recipient, you don't usually receive much information on your donor. All we knew after the transplants was the first heart was from a twenty-seven year old male from Las Vegas, Nevada and the second heart was from a nineteen year old male from Reno, Nevada. Both were the results of automobile accidents. We were informed by my social worker, Rodney Plante, that it was highly recommended to write a thank you letter to the donor of the second heart.

Once the letter was written, we were instructed to give it to the hospital where they would forward the letter on to the donor's family. If the family cared to respond to us, then they could do so. We never heard from the donor's family. Families often choose to remain anonymous due to the trauma over losing a loved one. However, maybe six months after returning home, we received a letter in the mail from the family who had donated the first heart. Evidently, they had contacted Stanford wanting to know who had received their son's heart. Understanding that I was the recipient, they wanted to know how their son's heart was doing. It broke our hearts having to write back informing them that their son's heart did not begin pumping after it was transplanted into my body. I mentioned how much we appreciated their true gift of love and because of their generosity, their son's heart allowed me to live long enough to receive a second heart and I was alive today in part because of their son.

16
Settling In

Mary

Thursday, August 17, was our best day and one we will both remember forever. When I got to Don about 8:00 a.m., he was already dressed and sitting up in his wheelchair eating pancakes. Not only was he eating, but he had finished almost half of his plate. Then at 8:30, I wheeled him downstairs to dialysis. On the way, we bumped into a man I knew from church. I didn't know his name, but every Sunday I sat behind him, his wife, and their young daughter. We chatted for a few minutes and I continued on with Don. A few hours later, when I was going back to pick Don up, I met the gentleman again. He stopped and asked me, "How is your father doing?" It took me a few seconds to realize he meant Don. I didn't know if I felt bad for Don because he had aged so much or thrilled that this gentleman thought I looked so young. I told him that my father had passed away twenty years ago and the man he just met was my husband, who was only four years older than me and was doing just fine.

After Don's dialysis, where they were only able to take off 1.8 liters of fluid, Evelyn, our social worker, explained all the drugs and appointment schedules. Next, Don got discharged out of the hospital to the apartments. Yes, he was actually discharged after almost 16 weeks at Stanford University Hospital. I wheeled him over to the Linx Restaurant on the Stanford campus. He didn't eat much, I think he was very excited and a little nervous. The Linx Restaurant is located walking distance from the hospital and was a change from the cafeteria food I had been surviving on for the past four months. So I ended up eating enough for the both of us. Don was so excited about getting to the apartment, but by the time I actually wheeled him over, got him upstairs, and he had a chance to look around, he was exhausted. Hence, he rested in bed while I put his things away and ran across the street to the Medical Pharmacy Plaza Drug Store to pick up all his drugs. I want to emphasize the word "all" because when I got to the pharmacy, they handed me a huge box filled with bottles, vials, syringes, and instructions. They were so patient with me, giving detailed instructions on how and when to administer the medications. Some had to be refrigerated and some had to be crushed with a mortar and pestle. I still had to buy a new blood pressure kit and scale because I had forgotten ours at home. I was petrified about being responsible for Don, but we made it through the first night. Best of all, he was able to use the bathroom almost totally by himself. I still placed pads under him and he wore diapers at night, but things were looking up.

Friday, August 18, was a pretty good day. He had slept through the night and told me it was one of the best night's sleep he had ever had. The home nurse came about 1:00 to set up a tentative schedule for physical therapy, since it was going to be at the apartment from then on. The rest of the day we sat by the pool and Don took a nap (in the shade) while I, of course, read a book. I still had questions about Cellcept and Gengraf; two of his anti-rejection meds, but I knew we could ask at his Monday clinic appointment at the hospital.

We set the alarm to have Don up, fed, medicated, and over to dialysis by 8:30 a.m. on Saturday August 19. He was finished and ready for me to take him back to the apartment by 12:30. Those three hours were great for me to get the place cleaned up, run errands, and even have time to listen to a murder mystery on my iPod. Having audible books to listen to all those months was a godsend for me. I do have to say, I received quite a few strange looks when I was listening to a Carl Haaisen book and burst out laughing all by myself. Two of the ladies at the apartments commented more than once about never seeing me without my earplugs plugged in. On this particular Saturday, I didn't do much listening after picking Don up because shortly after lunch, Mike came to visit. He was such a great help showing Don how to use the Direct TV upstairs on the third floor to watch the ball game. One thing that shocked both of us was Mike's new growth on his face. While he was in high school, he had bleached his hair blonde and now here he was with a dark beard. It took us by surprise, but it kind of grew on us. He also showed us his website for a new rock band he was in, called Guilty By Design. We were pleasantly surprised, it sounded very good.

After Mike left, we had a somewhat terrifying incident. Don was trying to get out of his wheelchair and up using the walker. I, in my infinite wisdom, had placed an area rug between the front door and the doorway to the bathroom. Don took one step out of the chair and slipped on the rug, falling completely to the floor. Well, I am a pretty strong person and Don only weighed about 112 pounds, so you would think, "No problem." I tried and tried to get him up to no avail. It was Saturday and no one was around. Anyone who would have been around, would be an invalid just like Don and would have been no use to me. But I started to panic and began knocking on each and every door in the building. I finally got to the very last door upstairs on the third floor at the very end of the hallway. When I knocked and waited, the door slowly opened and a huge, tall, football player type young man answered. When I explained my problem to him, he only asked how much Don weighed. I told him about 112 pounds and he said, "Okay let's go." He walked into our apartment, picked Don up like a 5 pound sack of potatoes, and said, "Where do you want him Mam?" He gently placed him back in the wheelchair and left. It all took about 5 minutes, but I was so extremely grateful. It turned out that he had been visiting a friend for the day who was going through a transplant and our timing was perfect. Later that evening, I baked some cookies and walked them up to him which made him very happy.

We had a pretty calm day on Sunday, August 20. Don was able to use the bathroom all by himself and get to and from with no assistance. He also took a walk with his walker down all the hallways on the second floor of the apartments. We tried getting on-line to order some airline tickets for a trip I was taking to Minneapolis. It was on the third floor because that was the only location in the building that our computer could get reception. We still had difficulty getting into Expedia.com and ended up doing it on the phone anyway. The reason I was taking a trip to Minneapolis was for a 40th high school class reunion. Nineteen of the twenty in our class were going to be there for the whole weekend. I was so excited, but at the same time I wondered if I would remember everyone's names.

* * * *

On Monday, August 21, Don had lab work at 8:15, x-ray at 8:30, clinic at 9:00, and an infusion for infection at 1:30. We both liked the clinic doctor, Dr. Hannah Valentine. She had a nice calm way about her. Plus I loved her shoes. However, it was a shock to both of us that there might be a need for this infusion every six weeks for quite a while. This was just one more issue to have to deal with. Don's blood pressure was high that day, but we were told that transplant patients usually tend to have higher blood pressure. That day they put him on two more new drugs; one was for cholesterol and the other was for blood pressure.

The next week was a busy one for both of us. Don had dialysis on Tuesday, Thursday, and Saturday. So on Saturday, August 26, although he started at 8:30 a.m., he didn't finish until almost 12:30. This all meant that after I got him back to the apartment, I had to give him his 8:00 a.m. meds at 12:30. It was doubly difficult because some of his meds he had to have one hour before eating, some with food, some he had to wait two hours after eating, and his Nepro had to be taken at 10:00 at night, and he had to remain upright for two hours before laying back down. We made a note to ask his nurse, Joan Miller from clinic on Monday, what meds he could take on dialysis mornings that wouldn't get flushed out during the process of dialysis.

The PT from Pathways ; an outside private therapy organization, named Barbara was wonderful. She came three day a week for an hour each time. She accomplished so much with Don and always left us with numerous exercises to practice, plus an upbeat feeling of hope that eventually Don would be back to his old self soon. On this particular day, she taught him how to go up and down the stairs with his cane (the collapsible one I had bought him for Father's Day.) She had him walking around the hallways holding on to the railings and then showed him how to get in and out of the car. On the Tuesday before, my nephew, John Jr. had sent Don a cane made from a bull's penis. It was three feet tall, the same length as the collapsible metal one, but it weighed so much more that Don was not able to maneuver it at the same time while trying to get his legs to work. However, it turned out to be quite a conversation piece when we did take it out or when people came over for a visit. They must have bigger bulls in Wisconsin!.

On Tuesday, August 29, Don had dialysis in the morning. They were late getting him started, but I was thrilled when I arrived back to pick him up three hours later because they had removed his pic line in his arm. This was also the day we started a new regimen of pill taking, one that was much easier to follow.

Although, I had been under a great deal of stress for the last four months, I must say that in some ways it had been like a mini vacation for me. I didn't have to go to work each day. I sat for three hours every other day during his dialysis reading or knitting. I didn't have to fix any meals for anyone but myself and I ate and slept when I wanted. The biggest plus was that until now I was only responsible for myself. That all changed now that Don was in the apartment with me. I worried constantly that I would make a mistake with his meds, that he would fall again, or that he would get another infection because I didn't clean his feeding tube correctly. My days were no longer my own and the nights were filled with fitful sleep over worry that he was so dependent on me and my limited skills. I stopped writing in my journal at night because I was usually so exhausted that I hit the pillow and was out for the count, only to wake up a few hours later fretting about the next day. It was a vicious circle;

not getting enough sleep at night, then so tired the next day that I couldn't wait to jump into bed at night.

We did have some fun times taking small excursions to the Rodin exhibit on the Stanford campus and a few trips to the Stanford Theater downtown to see movies. On one occasion to see Rodgers and Hammerstein's Oklahoma, I had to drop Don off in front of the theater so I could find a parking spot on a side street. When I walked around the corner of University Avenue, I saw Don sitting in the gutter begging people for help in standing up to no avail. He had fallen after getting out of the car and was not able to get his foot up over the curb. I understand that people are hesitant to get involved, but at the same time it was quite clear that he was too weak and in no condition to take advantage of a good Samaritan. Yet, no one would help him. I got him up, into the movie, and we did have a great time. However, from then on I never left him out of my sight.

On another impromptu mini vacation, we left after Don's Friday morning dialysis and drove up to our cabin in Tahoe Donner. We actually had a very relaxing weekend, just sitting on the deck being away from anything medical. When we got back for his Monday morning dialysis, his blood pressure was favorably lower.

17
Returning Home

Don

By the first part of October, I had mostly stopped using the walker and the wheelchair and advanced to using the cane. If we happened to be running behind for a scheduled appointment at the hospital, Mary would whisk me over in the wheelchair. Then, on the way back to the apartments, I would practice my walking. Even though my walking was rather slow and halting, I needed the practice while Mary worked on her patience.

During that early part of October, we were informed my release date from Stanford would be happening fairly soon. The nephrology department was in the process of getting me scheduled for my every other day dialysis treatments back home in Santa Rosa. Until placement was confirmed, we didn't have an actual date for going home. I had been cleared for my release from cardiology, but we had to be patient with our waiting to hear from nephrology. My new heart continued functioning wonderfully with no rejection. My appetite remained good and my weight had even increased to 117 pounds. Things were looking up! The home nurse and Barbara, the physical therapist, each signed off on my care and gave me their blessing for a long and wonderful new life.

While I was undergoing a dialysis treatment on the morning of Thursday, October 12, Mary rushed into the treatment room excitedly telling me she had received a call on her cell phone from one of the nurses, saying everything was in order for us to be released from Stanford.

Off she ran back to the apartments for packing up six months of accumulated gear into the SUV. She wanted to be ready to leave the minute I was finished with my session. That day was probably the most exciting for the both of us in the past many months. To this day, I don't know how Mary got everything ready in such a short period of time. She had our vehicle packed to the roof. I was surprised we didn't have stuff tied to the racks on top. We could have looked like the Beverly Hillbillies coming to California.

Wow, what an experience the past six months had been. We endured many highs and lows and frequent frustrations. Often, I questioned if I would ever be released from Stanford and if I was released, was I destined to spend the rest of my life in a care facility. But, with the wonderful care I received from the staff at Stanford and the love and support from family and friends, I somehow made it through. Having a fighting spirit and a personality type which perseveres, even when the odds appeared to be against me, were important factors. Most heart transplant recipients are able to return home in a matter of a few weeks after receiving a new heart, however I was at the other end of the spectrum.

At my release from Stanford, I was to return for scheduled periodic clinic appointments for biopsies, echocardiograms, blood testing, chest x-rays, and physician assessments with the cardiology and nephrology departments. My post-transplant cardiologist at Stanford, was usually Dr. Sharon Hunt. Follow-up visits at Stanford was something I had to be prepared for the rest of my life. Once again, I began seeing Dr. Hopkins in Santa Rosa in conjunction with Stanford visits.

Upon returning home, I had been scheduled for my every other day dialysis treatments at a facility in the town of Windsor, which was approximately a fifteen minute drive north of our home in Santa Rosa. Since my last treatment at Stanford had been on a Thursday, my dialysis days were to be Saturdays, Tuesdays, and then again on Thursdays. Three sessions a week every week for the rest of my life, or until I was ever lucky enough to somehow receive a new kidney. On dialysis days, we would get up by 5:30 a.m. and be at the facility in time to be hooked up to the dialyzer at 6:00 for my three hour run. The facility had a room of approximately forty feet square with maybe ten stations. Each station had a dialysis machine and an easy chair. The chairs were not too unlike recliners you might have at home. The room had a constant sound of hissing air as the machines performed their jobs of cleansing each patient's blood. Patients would either sleep, read, do word searches, or watch television while relaxing in their easy chairs during the three hour session. Since I wasn't allowed to drive as yet, Mary had to drive me there and then pick me up around 9:30 after I was finished. When I say finished, I was just that, finished. I had the strength of a wet noodle. The dialysis process made me feel limp afterwards; almost light headed, and I found walking difficult. So Mary would drive us back home, where I would lay down and rest for a while. After resting a couple of hours, I felt better and could resume the day. At the hospital and while at the apartments I didn't notice the after effects of dialysis as much, but trying to resume a more normal lifestyle after returning home became more of a challenge. Days in which I didn't have dialysis were much better days and I had a higher degree of energy.

My nephrologist, after returning home, was Dr. Benjamin Fritz, who had graduated from Stanford Medical School some years earlier and became involved in a medical practice in Santa Rosa. Upon being released from Stanford, my records had been transferred to his office where I was to be placed under his care. We met at one of my first dialysis sessions during one of his weekly visits to the treatment center. He would visit patients as they were being dialyzed, looking at their individual charts and answering any questions each patient might have. Dr Fritz was fairly young, had a friendly and gentle manner, and put each patient at ease. Knowing that Dr. Hopkins, Dr. Fowler, Dr. Oyer, and now Dr. Fritz, were all alums of Stanford Medical School, I felt I was a small part of an elite club.

Within a couple of weeks after returning home, I was able to stop using the cane and negotiating our stairs became much easier. My strength continued to improve each week, even with the minor setbacks on dialysis days. I had to be conscious of staying away from people with colds and flu. Early on, with my venturing about at Stanford and around the Palo Alto area after moving to the apartments, I was advised to wear a mask. So after returning home, I wore the mask for a short period of time. I needed to keep the odds in my favor for avoiding any new infections or viruses. When undergoing dialysis treatments for end stage renal (kidney) disease, the one substance that is not dialyzed out of a person's body is potassium. Because of that, the monitoring of potassium became very important. Again, I was to be challenged with yet another restrictive diet, not too unlike the many years of low sodium I had to follow before the heart transplant. Now my directive was to follow a low potassium diet. Like sodium, potassium is found in some degree in most foods and drinks. Dieticians at the dialysis center provided listings of foods and their contents of potassium. The easy part was studying the lists. However, staying away from the higher potassium foods took some effort. Some of the higher potassium foods I was instructed to stay away from, or have on rare occasions, and even then only in small amounts were; potatoes, tomatoes ,oranges, bananas, spinach, dark leafy green vegetables, milk, avocado, beans, and nuts. We were right back to reading labels and being as restrictive as we had with sodium. Will the fun ever cease? Potassium is a key element in diets for healthy people with healthy kidneys, but in patients with end stage renal disease, potassium could be viewed as a toxin.

Knowing that I had been successful with watching my sodium intake, I now knew I would do what was required to maintain a low-potassium diet. With Mary's diligence at the grocery store, we purchased foods that allowed me to sustain a fairly low-potassium intake. Grocery shopping became frustrating when dealing with so many diet constraints. Some examples of best choices for low potassium foods were; beef , chicken, and fish, cauliflower, corn, green beans, lettuce, onions, peas, summer squash, and zucchini, bread, cooked or dry cereal, oatmeal, muffins, popcorn, rice, apples, blueberries, cherries, fruit cocktail, grapes, canned peaches and pears, and their juices, coffee, tea, Crystal Light, lemonade, and lemon-lime soda.

Now, with a healthy heart, I didn't have to be quite as restrictive with sodium. But, because of the weakened kidneys, I didn't need to take chances of bringing extra fluid on board that my kidneys couldn't process. Since sodium can contribute to fluid retention, I was instructed to limit my liquid intake to around 32 ounces a day. The difficulty with those instructions were, that after returning home from dialysis, I could have consumed half of my daily allotment right then and there. Dialysis makes you feel very thirsty and dehydrated and the first thing you want to do is drink a gallon of anything you can get your hands on. Back at Stanford, I was always thirsty, but since I couldn't swallow, they could monitor my intake through the I.V. and with the lovely Nepro. Now, I was completely on my own.

I saw the importance of limiting my fluid intake when I would inquire at the end of my dialysis sessions of exactly how much fluid had been removed. Their response was, usually between 2 - 3 liters. A liter is closely equivalent to a quart. So the amount of fluid taken off in one session could be anywhere from ½ to 3/4 of a gallon. A gallon of water weighs approximately 8 pounds, so my 1//2 to 3/4 of a gallon would equate to 4 to 6 pounds per session. Before each treatment, I was weighed and then again at the end of the session. Usually my weight reflected at least a 4 pound loss. That was always a constant reminder as to how bad off my kidneys really were and the importance of limiting my fluids.

I noticed some patients weren't as diligent in regards to their diet and fluid intake as they should have been. Overhearing conversations with dieticians, nurses, and doctors, I could tell some diets weren't as closely followed as I knew I had to be with mine. Some patients were quite large and appeared to have other issues as well. I am guessing diabetes and high blood pressure might have been factors. It might be easy to feel that dialysis is going to clean your system and remove all the excess fluid. So on the non-dialysis days, you should be able to enjoy yourself. Right? Wrong!

Every week, each dialysis patient receives a report card of their most recent blood work, which is drawn during dialysis sessions. I felt good that my numbers were considered excellent. In fact, often being rewarded with gold stars at the top of the page, took me back to my elementary school days when you got your homework right or did well on a test. The potassium and glucose numbers were viewed as being very good for someone on dialysis. I guess those good numbers were enough incentive for keeping me on the right track with my diet.

After approximately a month at the dialysis center in Windsor, I was moved to another facility for my dialysis treatments. I had settled in nicely with the current situation, getting to know the nurses and patients that you see on an every other day basis. Due to staffing, scheduling changes, and patient load, it was necessary for some patients to be moved to a larger unit, which was located on the west side of Santa Rosa. Since my strength had improved enough, I had recently been released for driving and had become comfortable with the drive to Windsor. Now, my early morning drives were to be in another direction. The drive time was about the same as it was with going to Windsor, so my time schedule remained the same. When I said the new location was a larger facility, it was about four times larger and had approximately 44 dialysis stations. The machines and chairs were the same as I had experienced at the Windsor location and the room was maybe 40 feet wide by approximately 90 feet long. The facility was part of a large office complex which housed other offices as well as the offices of my nephrologists. With being a much larger treatment center, there was a constant transition of patients in and out of the unit for their 3 to 4 hour sessions. The entrance to the facility was often very crowded with buses and vans dropping off and picking up patients from local care facilities. Some patients had to be brought in on gurneys or in wheelchairs. I soon came to realize that I wasn't in all that bad of shape. At least, I could walk in for treatments and then walk out when I was finished and go about my day. Even though I was somewhat wobbly after a session, within a few hours that sensation mostly passed.

After experiencing treatments at Stanford, then back home in the Santa Rosa area, and seeing just how many people like me had to undergo weekly dialysis, I began to wonder just how wide spread kidney disease was. I knew of people who had experienced dialysis. In fact, my former father-in-law lived out his last years on dialysis. However, I never realized what a huge social and medical issue kidney disease had become in our world today. There are 485,000 people in the United States with end-stage renal disease and dialysis or transplants are the only ways to keep them alive. (National kidney Foundation (NKF), www.kidney.org.)   Over 92,000* people or roughly 80.7% of people in the United States who are waiting for organs, need kidneys. (U.S. Department of Health and Human Services (HHS), http://optn.transplant.hrsa.gov/data/. * As of April 5th, 2011.)

Amazingly, by the end of November, I was able to return to work and once again fulfill my duties as Vice President of Kresky Signs. I never knew if I would ever be in a position to work again. Most dialysis patients are unable to return to many of their former activities due to weakness, extreme thirst, headaches, fluid retention, and dietary restrictions. Only a little more than one-tenth of people on dialysis work either full-time or part-time. (NKF, www.kidney.org;

McGraw Hill Medical Text: Living Donor Organ Transplantation, 2008.) For many people, dialysis becomes their job. Although, I seemed to be one of the more fortunate ones. I am not saying that it was not difficult, especially on the every other day routine of dialysis. However, with my fighting spirit, I had a drive for trying to be more productive, rather than spending my life in a dialysis chair. Luckily, my job didn't have the physical demands as it had some years earlier and I could now perform my daily duties mostly at my desk. It felt great and satisfying having a purpose other than the constant dealings with medical issues. I worked five days a week. On non-dialysis days, I worked 8:00 a.m. to 4:30 p.m. On dialysis days, after returning home, I would have a late breakfast or early lunch along with 8 ounces of my closely monitored fluid choices. Those 8 ounces were always the most glorious substances to pass down my dry, parched throat. I would then rest for a couple of hours, which afforded me enough recovery time for making it down to work from 1:00 p.m. to 4:30 p.m. Returning home by 5:30, I knew I had endured a rather long day.

Continuing with intermittent catheterization remained a part of my daily program. At work, in a rather small bathroom, the process was always somewhat of a challenge. My set-up at home was quite convenient and precautions for keeping as sterile as possible were much easier. Performing the rather unpleasant task three to four times daily, I always equated the process as to what it might be like in preparing for surgery. The combination of anti-rejection drugs and the large diverticulum continued to be the perfect recipe for continued infections. Even trying to be sterile with the procedure, it was almost impossible for the avoidance of bacteria into the urinary tract. Adding the anti-rejection drugs and the diverticulum into the brew, I created the perfect storm for infections.

Taking urine specimens into the lab and being given a prescription for Cipro became fairly routine. The problem with that program was, if taken too frequently, you build up an immunity to antibiotics. With having the diverticulum on the bladder, it didn't allow the bladder to completely evacuate all the stored urine, thus making it easier for harboring infections. A solution to this was offered by a nurse in Dr.Palleschi's office. I was instructed to irrigate the bladder three times a day with a Neosporin irrigate and sterile water. After eliminating my urine with the catheter process, I would instill 50cc of the solution through the catheter into the bladder, holding it for 15 to 30 minutes before allowing it to drain. This process seemed to offer some success and the frequency of infections became less often. However, my next question was, would I need to perform this new task for the rest of my life? More on that to come.

The access for my three times a week dialysis was situated in a vein just below my right collar bone. It had originally been placed there, many months prior in ICU at Memorial Hospital, before I was transported to Stanford. At Stanford, the port had been relocated several times, and was now currently back in that same location. That type of dialysis access was not intended for long term use due to increased chances of infection. Now that it appeared I was probably going to be on hemodialysis for many years, a more permanent access was a better approach. Dr. Fritz's office set me up with a referral to see Dr. Douglas Green, a Santa Rosa vascular surgeon. Dr. Green's recommendation was the placement of an AV fistula (arteriovenous fistula), which is a surgical process of connecting an artery directly to a vein, usually in an arm. The fistula was to be the new access point for my dialysis. This procedure would create better blood flow during dialysis and was the best approach for long term use. It was recommended to perform the procedure as soon as possible because there would be some healing time involved before the fistula could be used. Also, it was important to get rid of the venous catheter sooner than later. Toward the end of my stay at Stanford, doctors had discussed the placement of a fistula, however, due to time constraints and insurance issues, the placement wasn't done at that time.

A surgery was scheduled for the placement of the fistula in my arm at Memorial Hospital. We arrived at admitting in outpatient surgery where we attempted to get checked in for the procedure. They took my blood pressure and temperature. Their findings were, that I had a fever. Because of having a fever, admitting said they didn't believe I would be able to have the procedure done at that time. However, they would call Dr. Green. He confirmed that I wouldn't be having any surgery until my temperature returned to normal. The problem was, surgery room scheduling was at a premium and it had taken a couple of weeks to secure the time which we now had to cancel. So we had no choice but to wait until I was fever free and infection free before attempting to reschedule, even though it might mean another few weeks.

I thought I was doing quite well with my dialysis routine and work schedule. However, Mary saw how much I struggled and how drained I appeared. Knowing that she was a universal blood type, Mary had offered to donate one of her kidneys to me when we were at Stanford. I said no at the time. Tara and Mike even offered to be tested. Again, I said no. I felt Tara and Mike were both too young and had their whole lives ahead of them. I didn't want them to possibly jeopardize their well-being later in life because of me. However, I was touched that they would even consider donating a kidney to me.

18
Testing For
Kidney Transplant

Mary

O ur days at Stanford continued with physical therapy, dialysis, and office visits consuming most of our time. Finally, on Thursday, October 12, 2006, after dropping Don off at dialysis, I returned to the apartment to tidy up and do some laundry. About thirty minutes into my chores, the cell phone rang. It was Joan from heart clinic telling me we were being released from the hospital. At first, I thought she was joking, then I screamed over the phone. I rushed back over to the hospital to relay the news to Don, then rushed back to the apartment to pack our vehicle with our of our belongings. I never packed so quickly in my entire life. Don was shocked when he saw the SUV and how much stuff I was able to cram in within a few hours. During the long drive to Santa Rosa, I was like a little kid on her way to Disneyland. I couldn't stop the euphoria.

When we arrived home, Don was fortunate enough to have been given a scheduled dialysis chair at a center in Windsor, a fifteen minute drive north of us. He was also able to keep the same schedule he had had at Stanford, of Tuesday, Thursday, and Saturday mornings. His time slot was from 6:00 a.m. to 9:00 a.m. We usually set the alarm for 5:00, got dressed, and arrived at the clinic at 5:45. They always took him right in. We never had to wait. Most days I just dropped Don off and returned home only to turn around to pick him back up between 9:00 and 9:30. It was extremely disheartening for me to see him after the three hours of dialysis. It was as if all energy had been drained out of his already compromised body. Don continually had a gaunt, yellowish grey skin tone. Later on a nurse told me the yellow color was due to the fact that the kidneys weren't able to process the urine properly and dialysis was only every other day. Sometimes, when picking him up from dialysis, I would have to actually put my arm under his and half carry him out to the car. I was so blessed that my school district had allowed me to take a leave of absence until December. I missed the work, but there was no way Don could have functioned on his own during this time. He would rally on his non-dialysis day only to return the next day to that weakened, drained condition. I realized that his ex-father-in-law had been on dialysis for over fifteen years, but I was positive that Don couldn't continue with this schedule for any more than a year or two. We had met many people at the dialysis clinic who were in the same boat as Don. Some were lucky enough to receive transplants, but those who weren't, slowly deteriorated before our very eyes.

Before we left Stanford, I had told the nephrology department that I was interested in donating one of my kidneys to Don. I had known from the very beginning, while Don was in ICU and the doctors had told us that Don would be on dialysis the rest of his life or would need a transplant, that I was a match. I am O positive and Don is AB positive. During all my years of donating blood at the blood bank, I had picked up enough information to know we were compatible. This only confirmed the fact that I had been telling Don for years that we were made for each other. So now, all I had to do was to be tested and convince the nephrology doctors that I was a good candidate and not too old to donate. At the first of the year, I went back to teaching full time, periodically taking off a day here and there to go back to Stanford for testing. I don't remember all the tests, but I do recollect twice having a urine test, where I collected urine for a whole day then took it to a lab to be analyzed. And twice, I had to wear a Holter monitor, because the first time they attached it to me we were staying overnight at a motel near the Stanford campus and must I must have pulled the leads out during the night. When we took it back to the hospital the next day, we were told there was no information on it and I would have to do it all over. A Holter monitor is a portable device which provides information similar to an EKG, with sensors attached to the body and to be worn for a 24 hour period. This device was very uncomfortable for trying to get a decent night's sleep.

Another test that I remember was one in which they called me to set up an appointment, but never informed me exactly what the test would be. Since I had been poked and prodded so many times, I didn't really think too much about it. Don and I drove down early one morning and showed up at the lab for our scheduled time only to be greeted with a very quizzical look from the attendant. I was dressed in a short skirt, top, and slip on heels only to be escorted into a room containing a treadmill and a heart monitor. I removed my shoes and even though I was barefoot, I performed very well.

Even the attendant was impressed. On the same visit, we had an appointment in Dr. Busque's office to explain the procedure more thoroughly with us and to have me answer some questions about my health and background. One of the questions was whether I was doing the donation for money. I looked at the nurse and said, "You better believe I am doing this for money. Don is going to be paying the rest of his life for this kidney. I see a lot of diamonds in my future." The testing went on from January through March or April when they finally acquiesced and allowed me to be Don's donor.

It was probably selfish on my part in wanting to donate the kidney because I saw how much Don was deteriorating and I couldn't bear to continue our lives like that. Did you ever have an instance where you witness a scene that pops up over and over in your head? I do. One day, shortly after Don had returned home after the second heart transplant and the months and months of rehab, he was standing in the bathroom facing the mirror. He had removed his clothes to take a sponge bath, since he still had the venous catheter in his right shoulder, right below the collar bone, and was asked not to get the site wet. I walked into the bathroom behind him and almost fainted. He looked like a Ethiopian refugee. His shoulders and hip bones were sticking out with two skinny sticks for arms and two skinny sticks for legs. I could count every bone in his rib cage, which resembled a skeleton with a thin layer of skin. Now, anyone that knows me can attest to the fact that I have always struggled with my weight, so you might think that I would be jealous of someone thinner than me, but he was just gross to look at. To this day, I still remember that image which haunts me and was the catalyst for assuring me I was making the right decision to donate.

19

The Kidney Transplant

Don

Sometime after the first of the year, 2007, on one of our clinic visits to Stanford., I was given the okay for a kidney transplant. After a physical and a complete health evaluation, it was determined I would be a good candidate for, yes, yet another transplant. But at the same time, my nephrologists at Stanford, Dr. John Scandling and Dr. Jane Tan, wanted me to wait at least year for recovery after the heart transplant before considering another transplant. If I was placed on a list for a kidney transplant, the wait time could have been 6 to 8 years. In 2010 over 4,700 people died on dialysis while waiting for a kidney that never came. (HHS, Organ Procurement and Transplantation Network, http://optn.transplant. gov/latestData/rptData.asp.) Mary questioned if I would even last the 6 to 8 years and was insistent that she be tested for being my donor. Even with her blood type being compatible with mine, her age of 58 at the time was a question in her eligibility for being a donor. Younger living donors are more preferable.

The winter and early spring months were filled with frequent trips back to Stanford for testing to see if Mary would be a good candidate. Now it was her turn to be poked, monitored, undergo CT scans, blood and urine assessments, EKG's, stress tests on a treadmill, and x-rays. However, there was something wrong with the new picture. Historically, over the last 16 years, Mary had stood guard over me with all my crazy health issues, and now it was my turn to watch over her. I guess turnabout is fair play and if Mary was to be my donor, thorough testing was required for her benefit and mine.

With our six month stay at Stanford for the heart transplants we became acquainted with many people. We were practically residents of the hospital with my unique situation and lengthy stay. So returning for clinic visits and now testing for a kidney transplant, we were frequently greeted in the hallways by staff inquiring as to my current health. When there are thousands of people in and out of Stanford Hospital and Clinics, on any given day, it's a warm feeling being remembered. We had almost been elevated to rock star status. Although, I don't know if that's the preferred way to attain notoriety, considering all that we had been through.

The times in which we did venture down to Stanford for Mary's testing were scheduled on my non-dialysis days. Stanford was very accommodating with scheduling appointments around my dialysis and our work schedules. However, this entailed awakening early so we could leave before the morning commute got heavy for our two hour drive. We never knew how much of the day our scheduled appointments would consume. On a couple of occasions we met for round table instruction and discussions with living donor coordinators from the Stanford Kidney Transplant Program. At these discussions we learned the particulars of what was involved with donating and receiving a kidney. Mary and I each received binders for study at home. It was almost a mini college course. The information covering the process placed us both more at ease as to what we might expect. Sometimes, after our day, we would leave the hospital before the evening commute and sometimes we would stay and enjoy a nice dinner in downtown Palo Alto, avoiding the commute all together.

Through discussions with transplant coordinators and doctors, we learned that there are two types of kidney transplant surgeries, a living donor which can come from a spouse, a family member or a close friend. The other type comes from someone who had died, which is referred to as a cadaveric donor. The cadaveric donor usually involves a long wait. So I was very fortunate we could consider the living donor approach which would be the preferred way.

By the end of April, Mary was approved for being my kidney donor. There had been some differences of opinions within the Stanford Nephrology Department as to Mary's future health after donating her kidney. Most all of her test numbers were good enough for being a donor. However, one kidney function test was considered to be borderline. They didn't want her to be faced with the possibility of kidney issues of her own later in life with having only one kidney. Taking chances of jeopardizing her future health also didn't ring well with me. After further discussion and more microscopic study of her kidney function, Mary was eventually given the okay.

I continued with a Monday, Wednesday, and Friday dialysis schedule , but hadn't been able to completely stay clear of infections. So we weren't able to re-approach the fistula surgery. During an office visit with Dr. Green, I brought him up to date with me being approved for a transplant at Stanford and that my wife Mary, was to be my donor. The fistula surgery was then placed on hold and I was instructed to notify him if anything should change with the planned kidney transplant. I was lucky that the current access port continued to provide proper dialysis and would hopefully do so until we were able to schedule the transplant.

We were eager to get the transplant scheduled, but we had to wait until Mary was finished with her school year which was sometime after the first part of June. Surgery was scheduled for Friday, June 22. We drove down the day before, got admitted to the hospital, and situated in our room to wait for more testing and analysis prior to the transplant. The two of us were able to share the same room. We had all the comforts of home, although we weren't allowed to share the same bed. Stanford was truly our second home, considering all of our visits and lengthy stays over the prior three years.

Our surgeon was to be Dr. Stephan Busque, whom we had met for consultations on a couple of prior visits. Dr. Busque was an associate professor at Stanford Medical School and his area of focus was kidney, liver, and pancreas transplantation. During these consultations, Dr. Busque explained what his approach would be with removing Mary's kidney and transplanting it into me. I remembered hearing stories of kidney transplants where ribs would be broken for both the donor and recipient. I guess at the time, this was evidently the needed approach in allowing for proper access to a kidney, which sounded almost barbaric and primitive. However, we were fortunate with current day medical advancements that Dr. Busque would be harvesting Mary's kidney through her abdomen. There was to be no incision, just a few small holes in her abdominal area, creating access for medical instruments to disconnect the kidney's blood supply and then the kidney's removal. As we learned, a kidney is mostly a network of blood vessels, and once the blood supply is taken away, the kidney becomes much smaller, maybe about the size of your thumb. The ureter, which is the passageway for urine from the kidney to the bladder, would also be disconnected. A sleeve would then be inserted through one of the holes, allowing for grasping around the now much smaller kidney, thus harvesting both Mary's kidney and the attached ureter. Sounds so simple, right? Well, probably not, but it certainly sounded less invasive than the breaking of ribs. Next, was to transplant Mary's kidney into me by means of another present day medical marvel. Instead of the rib breaking approach, my new kidney was to be placed in an area between my pelvis and right hip. There is a pocket in that location free of interference from other organs, which would accommodate the new kidney. Dr. Busque discussed in a very informative and understanding way, all that was involved with the harvesting and grafting of the kidney. This certainly made us more comfortable as what to expect. Of course, anything after the heart ordeal, would be a walk in the park. Dr. Busque would also be removing the bothersome diverticulum on my bladder that I had been contending with for several years and was a contributor to the many infection problems. Wow, someday I might be almost new. Dr Busque also mentioned that he would be leaving my original kidneys in their place. Although, they were hardly functioning anyway and weren't producing very much urine. However, the kidneys were to remain in place unless there happened to be issues with them down the road. I was also informed that my skiing days were probably over, due to the fact that the new kidney would not have any protection from ribs in its new location, and trauma to the area from a fall could lead to severe damage or even loss of the kidney. I said that I had given up skiing prior to the heart transplant and now that I was approaching 62 years of age, I didn't plan on skiing again, even though I certainly would miss it.

Prior to this most recent trip to Stanford, I had been struggling with a swollen right forearm and elbow. When Dr. Busque came into our room to discuss the transplant, I said we were both ready to get this done, but asked him to look at my arm. Upon examination of the arm, he said he could not perform the transplant with what appeared to be an infection in my body. I didn't know if it was the Ehlers-Danlos rearing its ugly head again. As a child, I would frequently get a swollen elbow or a swollen knee, which was usually the result of a contusion. However, in this most recent situation, I didn't remember knocking my elbow against anything. It was as though one day the swelling suddenly appeared. I suppose the swelling could have been a result of my overall weakened condition, dialysis, and the anti-rejection drugs. Hopefully, with the pending transplant, we would eliminate one of the culprits. So we had to head back home to get yet another infection cleared up. When we realized there wasn't to be any transplant the next day, I called the dialysis center in Santa Rosa from our hospital room making sure I would still have my chair available for Friday morning dialysis. I had informed the dialysis center sometime earlier that we had been approved for a kidney transplant, and that Wednesday, June 20 would be my last day for receiving dialysis. I was worried that my space would have been given to another patient due to the heavy demand at the facility. What would I have done then? However, they must have suspected I would be coming back, because of my infection problems. My chair was happily waiting for me.

Around the middle of July, and after several infusions, the infection finally cleared up. Dr. Fritz's office called down to Stanford and reported that I was currently free of any infection. The transplant was rescheduled for Wednesday, August 1. I am sure the thought was, "We had better get this guy down here and perform the transplant before anything else happens."

After not being able to have the first attempt at the transplant, I was hesitant in wanting to mention very much to my fellow dialysis mates that I had been rescheduled for the transplant. Besides, I felt uncomfortable that I was to be one of the lucky ones. I would now be able to get out of that place, lead a more normal life, and not have to depend on a machine to keep me alive. I am sure the other patients were very envious of my situation and yet I had complete compassion for theirs.

Another aspect I wasn't going to miss were the sponge baths and the tape jobs. The dialysis access point at my shoulder always had to be kept dry. Whenever I attempted to take a shower, Mary and I had to practically wrap my upper body in plastic and tape. It was such a long and labor intensive process that I opted to take a bath most of the time. The shower would have been my first preference, however the time involved hardly seemed worth the effort.

Mary's sister Ursie, from Wisconsin was scheduled to come out and take care of both of us after the first attempt of the kidney transplant. Of course, she had to cancel her plans and placed her airline tickets on hold until we rescheduled. Stanford would not allow us to be discharged from the hospital after the transplant until we had someone who would act as our care giver. We were fortunate again to be able to stay in the H.O.M.E. Apartments across from the hospital, just as we had after the heart transplant. Mary would not be in any condition for seeing to my needs and Ursie jumped at the chance to come to California to take care of us.

Tuesday, July 31, we drove back down to Stanford, repeating the same process as we had back in June. We even had the same room.

Although, this time I had no infection and everything was a go! After blood work and more pre-transplant testing for both of us, we anxiously awaited our big day. I don't think either of us had much sleep that night. We mostly just laid there and talked. Mary was taken to surgery at 6:00 a.m. the next morning to be prepped for the harvesting of her kidney which was planned for 7:00. I was taken later that morning for the transplant which was scheduled for noon.

While waiting in pre-op for surgery, our son-in-law, Spencer stopped by to wish us luck once again, as he had with the first attempt. He again was on a break from coaching. It was too bad he missed Mary, since she was still in recovery. The harvesting had gone well and Mary came through with flying colors. Now, it was my turn for completing the process. The only problem with the picture this time was that Mary wasn't by my side on the way to surgery, saying "Think Sex." But, I was a big boy, so I knew I could go it alone.

The next thing I remembered was waking up in intensive care with nurses around me, saying you have a new kidney and everything went very well. I looked over the side of my bed to see the catheter bag filling up nicely with light in color and crystal clear urine. A big difference compared to my kidney function after the heart transplant. I knew immediately, Mary's kidney, I mean my new kidney, was performing its designated job. I asked how Mary was doing and if I could see her? They informed me she was doing well and that I couldn't see her until the next day. I remember being extremely hungry because we hadn't been able to have anything to eat since the day before. They brought me a dry turkey sandwich, which I thought was probably the best turkey sandwich I had ever tasted.

Dr. Busque paid me a visit, explaining that everything had gone as planned. Mary's left kidney and ureter had been successfully transplanted in the pocket area to the left of my right hip. Dr. Busque also mentioned that he had removed the bothersome diverticulum on my bladder and was hopeful with its removal that my bladder would return to functioning normally. Wow, what a gift that would be. Mary and I had come through the process swimmingly and could expect many years of our kidney's functioning well together.

Thursday morning Mary was able to leave her room and come to visit me in intensive care. She looked great all dressed up in her new robe. You would have never known by her appearance of what she had experienced the day before. She was a little sore but otherwise felt great. After a visit to Mary's room later in the day, Dr. Busque felt she was doing so well that he would allow her to be released to the H.O.M.E. Apartments on Friday. Can you believe that? Donating a kidney on Wednesday and being released two days later. I even received the news that I would be moved to a regular room on Friday and if everything continued progressing well, I could be released on Sunday. What a turnaround from the heart transplant.

Ursie arrived in time on Friday to assist with Mary's release and take the two of them over to the apartments. She had flown in to Oakland International Airport where Tara picked her up then drove across the bay to Stanford. After getting settled at the apartment, Mary and Ursie walked back to the hospital to visit me in my new room. It was amazing to me that Mary could walk the one block each way after only the two days since donating her kidney. The marvels of modern medicine! Although, I strongly felt Mary's good Midwest German heritage might have been a contributing factor.

It was a good thing that my stay in the new room was to be only a couple of days because of all the crazy goings on in the bed next to me. There was a constant flow of people in and out of my roommate's bed area. He spent hours on the telephone. When he wasn't talking, he would be listening to loud music, even at night. He said the music helped him to relax. Hey, how about the other patients, or especially the guy next to him. I asked him to tone it down, but that didn't seem to matter. Consequently, I didn't get much sleep. So if I was to be discharged on Sunday afternoon, it wasn't going to be any too soon. I was amazed at how much better I felt so soon after the transplant. Even though I was quite sore, the pain killer pump that was attached to my I.V. was a big help in managing the pain. I guess I had become accustom to not feeling at the top of my game while undergoing dialysis for so many months. Now having a new and well-functioning kidney was a pleasant surprise. Dr. Busque was pleased with the results of my blood work and kidney function. We were informed the half-life of my new kidney could have been as much as twenty years. I said, "Sign me up for that." Twenty years would put me at 82 years of age. Who wouldn't go for that? Of course, they couldn't put that in writing. We also learned with time, the performance of one kidney could be as much as 60 - 70% of what two kidneys would do.

As was hoped, I was released from the hospital Sunday after-noon. Now I was able to join Mary and Ursie at the apartment for a couple of weeks of further recovery. When leaving the hospital, I still had a drain in the incision and a Foley catheter with a bag. Both were to remain in place for several more days while my body became use to all its new plumbing. The bladder needed time for healing af-ter removal of the diverticulum and the Foley catheter would allow for a continuous flow of urine. Now, it was a great relief knowing I didn't have to be concerned with the routine of undergoing dialysis every other day. Although, I wondered how all my former dialysis mates were doing?

Ursie had everything organized at the apartment, even down to numbering all my prescriptions so as to coincide with the number opposite each prescription that was listed in another binder that had been provided by the hospital. Again, I counted as many as 20 bottles or vials, which consisted of anti-rejection, anti-bacterial, anti-virus, and anti-fungal drugs. Also included were heart and blood pressure medicines that I had been taking since the heart transplant, as well as an assortment of vitamins. Ursie saw to the times for administering and the dosages for all medicines. Some were once a day, some twice a day, and one was three times a day. Ursie was our nurse, cook, and chauffeur. Mary and I don't know what we would have done without her excellent care and we will be forever indebted.

On one of our several clinic visits to the hospital during our recovery at the apartment, the Foley catheter and drain from the transplant incision were both removed. Without the Foley catheter, I would immediately know if I was to be able to regain the ability to urinate on my own. However, that was not to be the case. I thought with time and as the bladder healed from the removal of the diverticulum, my urinating would come around. Dr. Palleschi had informed me many years prior, that once you begin eliminating urine manually with intermittent self-catheterization, the bladder loses the ability to perform its designed function on its own. So I was back to performing the unpleasant task several times a day. However, the up side was, I had a great functioning, almost new kidney that produced some excellent urine.

Again we had visits from our children and grandchildren and along with Ursie it was like having a mini family reunion. We had some pleasurable dinners. Maybe they were even more so for me, knowing I didn't have to be as restrictive with my diet. This recovery period was drastically different from what we had experienced the year prior after the heart transplant. Having a new, healthy heart was now paramount in providing me with a much easier recovery period. There had been some discussion back at the heart transplant time, knowing most likely I would need a kidney transplant, of performing both a kidney and a heart transplant at the same time. On the other hand, they felt I was too weak to undergo both. I am thinking it was the right decision, because I probably wouldn't be here today, knowing I barely survived the heart transplant experience, let alone surviving a heart/kidney transplant.

20
Recovering From Surgery

Mary

Finally, around April or May of 2007, we received the long awaited phone call giving me the green light. Everything was set for June 22, which was a Friday. I was a little apprehensive because I had heard that more surgeries are botched on Fridays than any other day. But at the same time, I just wanted to get the whole thing over. When we arrived at the hospital, they put us both in the same room, which was wonderful. I had bought a new baby blue bathrobe and white slippers which I paraded around in. I listened to my iPod while lying around waiting for all the pre-op blood work and paper work. I had known that Don had a sore arm, but didn't think much of it until the doctor informed us there would be no transplant the next day due to Don's infection. My heart sank. Just then our son-in-law came into the room to visit us thinking he would be wishing us luck. At that time, he was working for the

Stanford football coaching staff and thought he would just pop in before going home that day. Don and I were so bummed, I never told Spencer how much we appreciated him coming to see us.

We drove home quite depressed, but resolved to the fact that we had to wait for Don's arm to heal. In retrospect, it wasn't a long wait. About the middle of July we got the okay from Don's nephrologist that he was healed and the transplant was set for August 1. So on Tuesday, July 31, we drove down and checked into the hospital. Both of us were so excited, we stayed up most of the night talking. Then about 6:00 Wednesday morning they came to get me for transport to pre-op. By 7:00, I was wheeled into surgery. I don't remember another thing until I woke up in my room. A very nice nurse was asking me how I was feeling. To be honest, I was a little sore in my abdomen, I felt hungry, but great! My only complaint I had about my stay was the other patient in the room who wined and complained all night about absolutely everything. So I didn't get a lot of sleep and the nurses wouldn't allow me to leave the bed to see Don until the next morning. They did tell me that he had done well during surgery and the kidney was functioning beautifully.

Early Thursday morning, after having a typical breakfast, they allowed me to walk down to Don's room in ICU. I was on the third floor and ICU was on the second floor. I had to gingerly take baby steps the whole way, but it was worth it to see Don sitting up, laughing with his nurse and Dr. Tan. He looked great and told me he felt even better. I stayed for a little while, then crept back to my room. Later that afternoon, Dr. Busque came in to see me and told me I could leave the hospital the next morning.

Very early Friday morning I was discharged then had to wait around for my daughter and sister to come and drive me over to the apartments, a block away. My sister Ursula had graciously rescheduled her flight from Wisconsin to stay and take care of us during our convalescence. They arrived early afternoon, picking up our car in the lot next to the hospital, and delivering me to the same apartments I had stayed in from June through October the previous year. This time however, we received preferred customer treatment and were given a larger unit on the quieter side of the building. Not only was the bedroom much larger, but there was enough room in the living room to accommodate a mattress for Ursie. She was a godsend. I don't know how we would have managed without her help and effervescent attitude about everything.

During our two and a half week stay, Ursie did all the cooking, cleaning, shopping for food, driving us to the Stanford Mall, and to The Ritz Carlton for lunch in Half Moon Bay. Many days we just sat around reading and resting. Other days she took us back and forth to the hospital for clinic visits. On Saturday, before we collected Don from the hospital, she drove me to Santa Rosa to pick up mail and get a few things from the house that we needed. It was a long drive and poor Ursie had to stop twice to allow me to use the restroom. When I asked Ursie later on what she remembered most about her stay, she said it was the trail mix she got at a Stanford Mall deli. It's funny the things we remember. I remember having terrible gas pains the first couple of days in the apartment until Ursie bought me a can of pears to eat. Cleared it right up! Besides being helpful, she was so funny. Once we tried to tell her how much we appreciated everything she was doing for us; cooking, administration of drugs, chauffeuring, etc. She looked at us and said, "This is the best vacation I've ever had." I replied, "How sad, you don't get out much, do you?"

21
Returning Home & BK Virus

Don

Mary and I had progressed so well with our recoveries that we were released to return home on Tuesday, August 21. It was so amazing to me that with only 20 days after receiving Mary's kidney we were allowed to return home, due in a large part to the wonderful care provided by Ursie. All my blood chemistry; (creatinine, potassium, etc.), and kidney function were considered excellent. We packed up all our gear and drove Ursie back across the bay to Oakland where she flew home to Wisconsin. I was instructed to return to Stanford in a couple of weeks for a follow up visit and blood testing, which was something I was certainly more than familiar with following the heart transplant.

After returning home, it wasn't long before we both returned to work. What an unbelievable feeling to be free of the chains of dialysis. Almost overnight, my whole being had been transformed.

I felt like that new person I had only dreamed about during the past few years. My appetite had returned and without being as restrictive with my food choices, hopefully my 120 something body weight would continue to increase. The only issue I now had to contend with was the intermittent catheterization.

With the healing of my incision, the kidney transplant scar is the one that I am probably the most proud of. The pencil line scar runs from just above the pelvic area across to the right hip bone. I am sure you think being proud of a scar is rather silly. Although, if you could see all my other war-like wounds from earlier years and the scars from a heart valve repair, two heart transplants, two defibrillators, and two hernia repairs, you might agree. Considering my Ehlers-Danlos Syndrome, I am surprised the incision healed so wonderfully. Dr. Busque performed a great job. I am often tempted to do a show and tell. Any woman would be so proud having a caesarian section scar as perfect.

Even with both of us back to working full time, we managed to take a few trips up to our cabin in the Lake Tahoe area for working on the landscaping around the property. I hadn't been in the best of form prior to the kidney transplant, so now having the strength to partake once again in more strenuous activities was simply marvelous. After many years, I had almost returned to my former self, thanks to loving and caring people and the marvels of organ transplantation.

By the fall of the year, we had settled back into a nice, comfortable program with our lives. Except to visit Stanford for clinic appointments and blood studies for the heart and kidney, our routine was mostly free of daily constraints in regards to my health. What a wonderful feeling. The holidays that year held an even more special meaning for being able to share enjoyable time with our children, grandchildren, family, and friends. After all, a couple of years earlier, my odds of being alive weren't that great.

However, sometime after the first of the year, 2008, my blood work assessments began to show an increase in the creatinine level. Creatinine is one of the key indicators as to how well kidneys are functioning. The creatinine level of my new kidney shortly after the transplant was 1.1 which was considered good. Healthy individuals with two properly functioning kidneys are at a reading of 1 or even a little under 1. A person with one kidney or a transplanted kidney might have a reading a bit higher, possibly 1.1 to 1.2. My level of creatinine began passing those, increasing to 1.3, 1.5, and as high as 1.7. Doctors Busque, Tan, and Scandling became immediately concerned that my new kidney was showing signs of rejection and a biopsy of the kidney was promptly performed by Dr. Tan.

With the new kidney so close to the surface of the skin, the technique for performing the biopsy was using, what looked like to me, a toy plastic gun which was placed on the skin directly over the kidney. Then with guidance from a monitor for proper location, a trigger type mechanism was pulled which allowed for retrieval of a tiny piece of tissue from the kidney which was then sent to pathology for study. After a couple of hours of waiting in a hospital outpatient room to make sure there was no bleeding, we were released to return home and wait for results, which could take a couple of days. The kidney biopsy was so much less invasive than I had experienced with heart biopsies where the access points are usually through the neck or groin.

The fun continues! After studies of the biopsy, blood work, and urine, it was determined I had what was referred to as a BK Virus. This is a virus that was first discovered in a kidney transplant patient in 1971 with the initials BK. This virus is thought to be in as high as 80 % of the population. The virus usually settles in the kidneys and urinary tract and lies dormant without any symptoms until a body has to deal with immunosuppression due to a kidney transplant and the subsequent taking of anti-rejection drugs. We don't know if Mary had the virus or if I had the virus or we both had the virus. Since we understood the virus was discovered in the Midwest, I tried to blame Mary. Just kidding! Anyway, none of that mattered, we now had to deal with treating the virus. A urinalysis showed I had millions of copies of the virus in my urine and if left untreated, the virus would eventually destroy my new kidney. So a very aggressive form of treatment had to begin immediately. If not, my future would be back in a dialysis chair. The choice of treatment by Dr. Tan was to have infusions of an anti-viral medication called Cidofovir. Initially the treatments were to be once a week. I would drive down weekly to Stanford for a three hour infusion administered with an I.V. in my arm. At each session, labs were checked, seeing how much improvement there had been compared to the prior visit. The Cidofovir proved to be very effective in fighting the virus. After three or four weekly visits, my schedule was changed to every other week. These sessions were not too unlike the hours spent in the dialysis chair, so to help in passing time more quickly, I would read, listen to books, and do word searches. By April, with Stanford's aggressive approach, the virus was gone. We were fortunate the virus was cleared up in rather short order because a side effect of using Cidofovir can cause toxicity to the kidney. The downside of contracting the virus was that my new kidney's function became somewhat compromised. The virus had slightly impaired the ability of the kidney to perform its designed purpose to the extent that was intended. Even though the virus was gone, my creatinine level continued to increase. Dr. Tan thought the best reading we could expect was a level at something around 2.0. I wasn't aware of any physical signs that my kidney wasn't performing quite up to par. The volume, color, and clarity of the urine was the same as it had been right after the transplant. However, as before the transplant, I continued with numerous urinary tract infections. We spent the best part of a year having lab tests for blood and urine, then being put back on a program of taking Cipro. During this time, Stanford was adjusting my Prograf dosage, trying to find the proper balance where my blood level of the drug was high enough to ward off rejection, but at the same time low enough to prevent the constant infections. When these infections occurred, my urine became cloudy and the creatinine level would spike up to as high as 2.4. So with the Cipro and a slight downward modification in the dosage of Prograf, after a couple of weeks, the infection cleared up and the creatinine reading was back at a level of around 2.0. If there was any good part to all of this, I was setup with a local lab in Santa Rosa that would send my results down to Stanford rather driving two hours each way for testing.

It wasn't until sometime in 2009 that I finally was able to move past all the infections and the constant adjustments to the immuno-suppression drugs. Finding that perfect balance in the daily dosage of Prograf seems to have kept me infection free. Currently, every three months I have a complete blood work-up, either in Santa Rosa or at my every six month visits for the heart at Stanford. As of this writing, I am holding my breath, but I haven't had a urinary tract infection in the past three years and the dosage of drugs has remained unchanged. Plus, Stanford nephrology says that I am doing so well that it is not necessary to see them any more than once a year unless they notice any changes. I consume a fair amount of water on a daily basis which allows the kidney to stay well hydrated. I continue limiting the consumption of potassium which keeps those numbers within accepted areas and the creatinine reading seems to have leveled off at a baseline of 2.0. Finally, after many years, my body might be back in balance.

If Mary had known the ride she was in for when we first met almost 28 years ago, she could have easily said, "I am out of here!" If I were to live two lifetimes, I would never be able to repay Mary for what she has done for me. It wasn't enough being by my side all the years while I struggled with congestive heart failure and seeing me through two heart transplants. She then offers me the true gift of love with the donation of her kidney. How do you top that? I know that I am the luckiest man in the world for having Mary as my wife.

22

So Thankful

Mary

Don and I were discharged from the apartments on August 21. Although we didn't have a lot to pack up after three weeks, Ursie did most of the loading into our car and we then drove her to Oakland International Airport. From there we went home, which never looked so great. We settled in that weekend and I returned to work on Monday. I was sore, but managed just fine. People would ask me how difficult it was to give a kidney and I still to this day reply that it was a piece of cake. I have had a ruptured appendix, two caesarian sections, a frozen rotator cuff, and I still say the kidney transplant was the easiest surgery I've ever had. I must say that my stomach looked like a relief map of the United States after all those surgeries, but Dr. Busque did an excellent job with the kidney surgery. There are just three teeny, tiny scars that you have to stare to find. Dr. Busque once asked me before the surgery if I would mind that I would probably not want to wear a bikini afterwards. I told him I never wore a bikini before. Why start now? Everyone at school that asked to see my scars were amazed. This usually lead into my campaign for others to put their name in for organ donation. I only wish I could convince more people of the good they can do for others, but also the good it does for them to know they can change someone's life with the most thoughtful gift on earth. And it's free. It doesn't cost the donor a cent. The recipient's insurance usually picks up the entire cost. Well, that's my plug for organ donations.

By September, Don was also back to work full time and we both settled back into a comfortable routine, minus his trips to dialysis three times a week. Then sometime in the middle of September, I called Chris Smith, who writes for the local newspaper. It was an odd request, but I was hoping he would put an article in his column thanking the numerous people who had supported us throughout our ordeal. We had people who watched our house, sent cards, phoned on a regular basis, and often made the long drive down to visit while Don was unconscious and during the many months of recovery. Chris asked to talk directly to Don, so I gave him Don's work number. It turned out that after talking to Don, he wrote the article mostly about the fact that Don received the kidney from his wife. So I would like to here and now thank each and everyone who stood by and supported us all those months before the transplants, during our stays at Stanford, and the many months afterwards.

Since then, both Don and I are doing swimmingly well. Plus, for about four years after the kidney transplant, I was in a study group conducted partly at Stanford to track the progress of kidney donors and how well their remaining kidney is functioning. For my age group, I was told I was doing very well and that my kidney was functioning at 68% of two. I personally wouldn't even know I had given a kidney except that I have some tiny scars and I have become a cheap date. After a glass or two of wine, I feel the alcohol go right to my head which was definitely not the case before the transplant. Other than that, our lives are healthy, full, and ecstatic that we have each other. Although, we have had some bumps and curves on our road together, I know we are blessed to have one another. We appreciate each and every moment we have and hope that with a new heart and a new kidney, Don and I will have many more years together, hopefully with no more transplants.

23
New Beginnings

Don

In the past, I have heard that recipients of transplanted organs can take on certain traits of their donors. I my particular situation, I haven't noticed that to be the case. I don't feel that I am any different now than before the transplants. I don't think I am any smarter or dumber. However, I am probably still anal, maybe even more so. Mary will say to me, "Don, your anal is showing." I always turn around and never see anything, but I am sure Mary is probably right.

With all my transplants, I have become much younger. I figure I now have a new average age. My new heart is currently 25 years old. Mary's kidney (my new kidney) is 64 years old, and I am 68 years of age. So now, I calculate that my new average age is 52. How can you beat that? While everyone is getting older, I have become 16 years younger. I guess I have discovered my own version of The Fountain of Youth. Even though, I wouldn't recommend my route as the desired choice. There is not a day that passes without remembering just how fortunate I am to have been blessed with being the recipient of donated organs. I most likely would not be here today if it wasn't for the love and generosity of others.

When I first began thinking of writing the history of my medical experiences, another title that came to mind was The Magic of Three, because the number three seems to have repeated itself many times throughout my life. I am the third Don in my family, named after my father and grandfather. I am the oldest of three children. Mary is my third wife. Together we have three children. We have three grand-children. I've had three hearts and I have three kidneys. I use to think my lucky number was number seven. I haven't figured out what the meaning of the number three phenomenon is, but if nothing else, three has to be my new lucky number.

Talking about lucky numbers, another number I constantly worried about was the possibility of surpassing the five million dollar cap on my health insurance coverage. At one point I recall being over three million and that was before the kidney transplant. Also, my coverage paid for all of Mary's hospital related expenses for being the donor. So I was petrified that we might have to incur some big time out of pocket expenses. As it turned out, we were close to the cap but were able to stay under the five million dollar figure. Thanks for wonderful health coverage! I may not quite be The Six Million Dollar Man, but I am certainly close to it.

Mary and I both retired from our jobs in 2010. Mary retired at the end of May after working twenty-eight years with Santa Rosa City Schools and I followed in July, retiring as president after twenty-eight years at Kresky Signs, Inc. Mary and I are still major stock holders in the company while I sit on the board of directors and assist as needed. With transplant recipients, it's never known how many years might lie ahead, so we wanted to allow time for enjoying each other, our home, children, grand-children, and travel. In the past year, I might have somewhat redeemed myself in the area of cancelled vacations. Since our retirement, we've spent our 25th anniversary in St. Martin and finally took that long awaited cruise.

Since my heart condition lead us to our first trip down to Stanford University Hospital and Clinics some eight years ago, we probably have made close to one-hundred trips. That's a lot of time, money, and miles. Of course, none of that matters compared to the degree I have received in continued living. Most people who choose to attend Stanford work toward a degree in law, medicine, finance, etc. I guess I followed a different path.

In the last three years, my health program has certainly stabilized. Currently, I have only two visits a year at Stanford with Dr. Hunt, one in nephrology with Dr. Tan or Dr. Scandling, two visits with Dr. Hopkins, and blood tests every three months. Presently, heart biopsies are not being performed on me. Echocardiograms (ECG) are done at the six month visits to Stanford and angiograms are performed once a year. There is now a new procedure for performing angiograms, where access to the heart can now be provided through the wrist which is much less invasive than through the groin. Quicker recovery time is also a major benefit. Periodically, I have appointments with Dr. Palleschi for prostate checks and plumbing issues and I continue today, as I will the rest of my life, dealing with my bladder function. I don't leave home without my catheter supplies. I also see a gastroenterologist and a dermatologist. People who have had transplants are at higher risk for developing skin cancers. So it is very important to be aware of any changes on the skin and have check-ups at least once a year with a dermatologist. Once again, immunosuppressant drugs are the offender. While warding off rejection, the use of anti-rejection drugs can hinder the ability of the body's immune system to repair UV damaged cells. This in turn can cause those cells to develop into cancers. I am very aware of sun exposure and continue the use of UV protection whenever I am outdoors.

What does the future hold? Implantable mechanical kidneys are now in developmental stages and could someday be an option to dialysis and/or having to wait on a kidney transplant list. And who knows where the future might lead us with stem cell research and how that might play into treatment of heart disease.

Having appointments over the years with Dr. Palleschi and his awareness of all my health issues, he has compared me to the Eveready Rabbit. On several occasions, he has said to me, "No matter what life has thrown at you Don, you always get right back up and continue on." I guess he is probably right. I do keep coming back. You can't quit. I always felt I had to hang in there, never giving up. Life is full of challenges and besides, where does giving up get you? Keeping a positive attitude and knowing there is something better down the road will carry a person a long way. I've had people tell me that I am the toughest guy they know. Physically, I am far from that. The toughness comes from my inner strength. Although, my weight has now increased to 145 pounds, this is a far cry from the 103 pounds after the heart transplant. I guess frequent trips to the gym for light work-outs and a good diet have shown some results. With all the health issues I have confronted over the many years, I feel fortunate I am still here today and able to pass on my story with its happy ending. Maybe I am the cat with nine lives. I hope this writing helps others that might be or have been faced with similar issues and realize that with keeping a positive attitude, having the wonderful care of great doctors, nurses and technicians, and the love and care of a fantastic wife, children, family, and many friends, there can be a better life out there.

www.ingramcontent.com/pod-product-compliance
Lightning Source LLC
Chambersburg PA
CBHW030434290526
45786CB00001B/287